Contemporary
Practical/Vocational Nursing

Corrine R. Kurzen,
MEd, MSN, RN

Coordinator, Practical Nursing Program
School District of Philadelphia
Philadelphia, Pennsylvania

D0910652

J. B. Lippincott Company   *Philadelphia*
London   Mexico City   New York
St. Louis   São Paulo   Sydney

Acquisitions Editor: Patricia L. Cleary
Designer: Susan Hess Blaker
Editorial Consultant: D. J. Arneson

6   5   4   3   2

Library of Congress Cataloging-in-Publication Data

Kurzen, Corrine R.
  Contemporary practical/vocational nursing.

  Includes bibliographies and index.
  1. Nursing   I. Title   [DNLM: 1. Nursing.   WY 16 K96c]
RT42.K87   1989   610.73   88-13186
ISBN 0-397-54715-3

. . . to good friends, for their love and encouragement

Preface

This book is intended to provide part of the foundation of your career in practical/vocational nursing. Each chapter has a specific focus designed to introduce you to the foundations of contemporary practical/vocational nursing.

Suggestions on how to adjust to being a student and how to develop good study skills will help you organize your self and your time. Discussions of the importance of maintaining a balance between your personal life and your academic and clinical life will help you develop and maintain good mental health practices. A study of the history of nursing will give you a sense of your heritage and your future. An overview of practical/vocational nursing education will help you recognize and adjust to your role as a student. A review of some of the nursing theories and the nursing process will introduce you to how patient care is implemented. An explanation of the health care system will help you understand how health care is delivered in the United States. A review of the types of health care facilities and the patient care team will introduce you to the variety of facilities and people who provide patient care. You will explore the differences in humankind and recognize the reasons for approaching each person as a unique human being. You will become acquainted with ethical issues in health care, and you will learn how to practice nursing within the law. You will have a brief overview of leadership, management, and organizational membership. Hints to help you as you begin your career will be offered. Current issues, future concerns, and continuing education will complete your introduction to the practical/vocational nursing career.

Your decision to become a nurse will undoubtedly change your life. The experiences you will have will expose you to the sorrows and the joys of being human. You will acquire knowledge and learn nursing skills, but beyond that, you will learn how to care effectively.

Although our contemporary society does not place a lot of value on providing services or on "caring" for strangers, you have chosen a career that requires both. Your special ability to care and provide care for others will be appreciated by the hundreds or even thousands of patients you will serve during your practical/vocational nursing career.

Your faculty has designed an instructional program that will take you from where you are now to being a nurse—a process that is often challenging. You will spend many hours studying and preparing for clinical assignments. You will experience joy and frustration. You may occasionally wonder whether the effort is worth it. But you will persevere, and you will succeed because you have a special ability to care for others.

It is my hope that you will continue to care as much as you care today. Take pride in what you do and how you do it, and treat all people with dignity and respect. You will feel a tremendous sense of self-satisfaction that comes when you know you have done your best.

Author's Note

I recognize that there are an increasing number of men in nursing, and I encourage and welcome their entering the field. However, for the sake of clarity and convenience, I have continued to use the feminine pronoun, except in a few instances, when referring to the nurse and the masculine pronoun, in most instances, when referring to the patient. These pronouns have no other significance.

Acknowledgments

I would like to thank the following individuals for their review and critique of the manuscript:

Janet M. Carpenter, RN, MEd
Supervisor
Health Occupations, Choffin Career Center
Coordinator/Director
Choffin School of Practical Nursing
Youngstown Public Schools
Youngstown, Ohio

Helen C. Harrell, RN, MS
Director
Herman School of Vocational Nursing
Houston, Texas

Mary Pauline Hurlburt, RN, BSN, ME
Former Coordinator
Tulsa Area Vo-Tech Practical Nursing Program
Tulsa, Oklahoma

Elizabeth V. Moore, RN, EdS
Director of Health Occupations Programs
Middlesex County Vocational/Technical Schools
112 Rues Lane
East Brunswick, New Jersey

Ruby O. Wang, RN, BSN
Practical Nursing Instructor
Emily Griffith Opportunity School
Denver, Colorado

I also extend special thanks to Patricia Cleary, Senior Nursing Editor, whose determination to see this book become a reality exceeded my own.

Contents

1 Adjusting to Student Life

Objectives

When you complete this chapter, you should be able to:

Design a schedule that includes time for study, personal needs, and family, social, and recreational activities.

Describe your role in learning through lectures, audiovisual presentations, computer-assisted instruction, and reading assignments.

Organize your notes and notebooks according to subjects and dates.

Use dictionaries, as well as tables of contents and indexes in textbooks, to find specific information.

Find information in the library by using the card catalogue, the services of the librarian, or both.

Use test-taking skills when taking various types of tests.

Explain the relationship between classroom and clinical instruction.

Twenty-three women and men ranging in age from 19 to 53 years became suddenly silent as Mary Henderson entered the classroom. Mrs. Henderson, a registered nurse for "more than 20 and less than 30 years," as she liked to say, walked briskly to the front of the room. She was a handsome woman with a proud bearing that reflected her feelings about herself and her profession.

"I'm your instructor," Mrs. Henderson said with a serious look. "We'll be spending most of the next year together, much of it right here in this classroom. I won't apologize for the age of the building. I'll only say that both of us have seen our share of eager students enter—and more classes graduate than either of us would like to admit." She smiled brightly. The class responded with a laugh. Mrs. Henderson surveyed the students, face by face. "There are 23 of you in this class today," she continued. "How many of you expect to be here when we assemble on graduation day?"

The room became silent. The students looked around the room at one another. Slowly, 23 hands went into the air. Mrs. Henderson nodded approval. It was exactly the kind of confidence she liked in a new class. She had a good feeling about this group. The students' positive attitude was already beginning to show. She knew it would be invaluable later when they would be deep into their studies and might need a boost through the hard work that lay ahead.

"And how many think the others in this class will be here with you when you graduate?"

Every hand shot up without hesitation.

"Wonderful," Mrs. Henderson exclaimed. "That's exactly what I had hoped. And that's exactly the way it will be if we all work together to stay together. However, it's possible that some won't be here to graduate. I frankly doubt it, with such an enthusiastic group as this, but it could happen. The decision will be yours." She paused. "Every one of you has the potential to succeed in this program. You wouldn't be here if you didn't. And I would not be here if I didn't have faith in you, too. It won't always be easy. But I know the goal is worth it because I've been a nurse for . . ." She smiled. "I almost said how long, that time, didn't I?" The class laughed.

Once again Mrs. Henderson looked into the face of each of her students. "All right, class. We've made our decision. I, your program, and the administration will do everything we can to support that decision. We're all in this together to become nurses. Let's get to work to make it happen." The students broke into spontaneous applause. Now they were a class.

Your decision to become a licensed practical/vocational nurse can be one of the most fulfilling choices of your life. In one year you will be ready to enter practice. The knowledge and experience you gain in that year will prepare you for an important career that is valuable to society and personally rewarding.

The months ahead will be full. You will work on a busy daily schedule with new ideas, information, and people. You will be asked to make hard decisions. When asked to do something, you will be expected to do it. Much of what you do will be influenced by rules and regulations. In addition, you will have to balance the demands of your personal life with those of your student life. How well you adjust and learn will become the foundation of your career.

But you have been a student before. Whether that was last year or years ago, being a student again is not a totally new experience for you. Being a student nurse will take hard work and dedication, but you have made the first step already. Your program will prepare you for the rest.

Orientation

Student orientation sessions with faculty and staff are held early in practical nursing programs to familiarize new students with their program's facilities and hospital affiliations. In them the rules and regulations for class, hospital, and residence conduct are explained. The program's courses and course content are described. If there is a student government, it is explained.

Information about important student services, such as library, health, and counseling services, is given in detail.

The more you know about your program, its requirements, and what is expected of you before the program is fully under way will make a big difference in your success as a student. Student orientation sessions are the perfect times to ask questions. If you have already had your student orientation, review the information you were given. If you have more questions, now is the time to ask an instructor for the answers.

Adjusting to Student Life

Adjusting to student life requires more than knowing rules and regulations, and it is more than studying and learning. *Self-awareness*—being conscious of your own feelings and how well you fit in—is equally important, and we'll discuss this in depth in Chapter 2.

Caring for others is a big responsibility. It is often demanding. Your program is preparing you to give nursing care to your patients. The better you understand yourself, the better that care will be.

Understanding oneself improves the quality of the care given because full attention is on what has to be done, without interference from personal issues. If you cannot take care of yourself, your effectiveness as a nurse will diminish.

Taking care of yourself means to be aware of, to understand, and to provide for your own physical, emotional, and intellectual needs. These needs may be complex or simple.

Being aware of your needs and what to do about them is your responsibility. But you are not alone. Your instructors and program administrators know that personal, social, and scholastic problems can arise at any time.

Counseling services to help students make adjustments and solve problems may be available to you. Make use of them. If your program does not have special counseling services, discuss your needs with your program advisor, your instructors, or other members of the faculty or administration. Don't hesitate to ask for help or advice—the sooner, the better.

Your Program

Organization and Curriculum

Your program may vary somewhat from other practical nursing programs, but the foundation of most programs is similar. In general, they present basic nursing and health care theory and principles in classroom lectures.

Clinical instruction is provided in a hospital, nursing home, or community health facility.

Programs are approximately one year long. Some are sequential, with classroom instruction followed by clinical instruction. Others offer a concurrent curriculum, which presents theory at the same time as the clinical rotation in that subject. Programs are usually sponsored by junior colleges or vocational/technical schools in affiliation with hospitals or health care institutions.

Basic course curricula for programs include communications, anatomy and physiology, pharmacology, professional adjustments, contemporary health issues, fundamentals of nursing, sociology, psychology, mathematics, geriatrics, nutrition and diet therapy, maternal and child health, and medical-surgical nursing. Cardiopulmonary resuscitation (CPR) and first aid courses may also be required.

Program Structure

Your success as a student will be improved if you understand and use your program, its organization, and its personnel efficiently. Each part of your program has an objective.

Your school's objective is to provide an organized curriculum—required courses—to pass the licensing exam in your state for practical/vocational nurses.

Your instructor's objective is to teach you the information in the course.

The administration's objective is to manage the program so that all other objectives are met.

Learn why your program is structured the way it is. Find out why each course is included. Ask what you are expected to do. Much of your success will depend on how well you prepare. If you know what to prepare for, doing what is expected will go smoothly.

Get to know your institution and its administration. Learn who the people are who run it. Find out what they do. The information will be invaluable when you need help.

Know your instructors. Find out what they expect of you. Learn their views on class discussion. Knowing who welcomes discussion and who prefers to lecture without interruptions tells you when to ask questions and when to be a good listener. Find out how your instructors feel about their relationships with students. Some may like open, friendly associations. Others might prefer well-defined lines between teacher and student. When you know your instructors' preferences, you can avoid the mistake of trying to warm up to someone who views such friendliness as improper.

Familiarize yourself with the importance of grades, quizzes, and tests. Find out how tests are scored and which count more than others. Learn the value of class participation, homework, punctuality, and attendance. Ask whether typed papers are preferred over handwritten papers.

In other words, learn everything you can about your program and the people in it. The more familiar you are with your program, the easier it will be to adjust to it. Your immediate objective is to integrate your student life with your personal life so that you can concentrate on your long-term goal— to become a licensed practical/vocational nurse.

Scheduling Your Time

How you use your time can make the difference between being prepared and falling behind. Almost every day will be full. On occasion, you may wish there were more than 24 hours in a day. Finding the time to get everything done may take some ingenuity. And when you do find extra time, you'll treasure it. A written schedule is a good way to organize your time to put every hour to its best use.

A good schedule should be realistic. To get the most out of your program and still have time for your personal life, make a schedule that fits the time you have, not how much you wish you had. Set your tasks and the amount of time to do them according to what you can reasonably expect to get done.

Use your class schedule as the basis for organizing the rest of your time. A well-organized schedule should let you see a full week, hour by hour, at a glance. For a sample schedule, see Table 1-1.

The easiest way to schedule your time is to buy a pocket- or purse-size calendar made especially for the purpose and use its organization as the basis for your own daily and weekly program.

Learning Methods

Learning and Intelligence

Simply defined, learning is acquiring knowledge, skills, or attitudes. How well one learns depends on the ability to study, the motivation to learn, and thinking, reasoning, and problem-solving skills. Evidence of learning can be observed in or through changed behavior.

Intelligence can be defined as the ability to adapt what one knows to new situations. Put another way, how easily one can solve problems is a measure of intelligence. Intelligence is a combination of memory, imagination, acquired knowledge, and judgment. It is partly dependent on what you already know and partly under your control to change.

Intelligence also reflects one's heredity and environment. Heredity is

Table 1-1.
Typical Week-Day Schedule of a Mother With Two Children

	Monday	Tuesday	Wednesday	Thursday	Friday	Saturday/Sunday
5:30	Get up, shower and dress, breakfast					Sleep
6:30	Drop children off at babysitter					Get up and dress
7:00	Travel to school — Memorize math equivalents on flash cards					Study Math
8:00	Anatomy class	Anatomy class	Anatomy class	Anatomy class	Anatomy class	Shopping and household chores
8:50	Anatomy class	Anatomy class	Anatomy class	Anatomy class	Anatomy class	
9:40	Psychology class	Psychology class	Psychology class	Psychology class	Psychology class	
10:30	Break	Break	Break	Break	Break	
10:40	Nursing class	Nursing class	Nursing class	Nursing class	Nursing class	
11:30	Review lab procedures	Review for math test	Make flash cards	Review lab procedures	Meet with advisor	Recreation
12:30	Nursing class	Nursing class	Nursing class	Nursing class	Nursing class	
1:20	Math class	Nutrition class	Math class	Nutrition class	Nursing class	
2:10	Vocational Relations class	Sociology class	Vocational Relations class	Sociology class	Math class	
3:00	Travel from school — Memorize medical terminology on flash cards					
4:00	Pick up children from babysitter					
4:30	Household chores; dinner with children					Household chores
						Dinner
6:00	Study Nutrition	Study Math	Study Nutrition	Study Math	Study Vocational Relationships	Recreation
7:00	Study Anatomy	Study Anatomy	Study Anatomy	Study Anatomy	Study Anatomy	Study Psychology
8:00	Study Nursing	Study Nursing	Study Nursing	Study Nursing	Study Nursing	Review all notes from past week
9:00	Study Sociology	Study Psychology	Study Sociology	Study Nursing	Study Psychology	Relax
10:00	Relax	Relax	Relax	Relax	Relax	Sleep
10:30	Sleep	Sleep	Sleep	Sleep	Sleep	Sleep

what you're born with and can't be changed. Environment is the condition you live in and can be changed.

An ideal learning environment is one where one's whole attention can be directed to learning. Such an environment is unrealistic because life, for most people, is filled with a variety of interests and obligations that compete for time and attention. However, you can change the parts of your environment that interfere with your studies. Identifying them and changing them will improve your ability to learn.

Lectures

The backbone of your program is your classroom lectures. They will be the basis for everything else you do. Most of what you will be expected to learn will be given first by your instructors in classroom lectures. The classroom is where you will be informed of what is expected of you. It is where you will have the best opportunity to ask questions. How much you get from lectures will depend on how good a listener you are.

Listening

Listening and hearing are not the same. Hearing is biophysical. It is perceiving sounds. Listening is intellectual. It is a conscious effort to hear. You may hear what someone says but not know what is meant. To understand something requires listening. In lectures and elsewhere, listening takes effort.

Being a good listener is one of a nurse's most useful skills. Throughout your career, most of your interactions with instructors, other nurses, physicians, and patients will be verbal. Even the observations you make will depend heavily on what you hear as well as what you see. Knowing what is said can affect how well you perform.

To listen effectively, fix your eyes on the lecturer's face. Pay close attention to the words, following them in your mind. Make your written notes while you listen, but concentrate on what you're hearing rather than on what you're writing.

Taking Notes

Nobody is expected to remember everything he hears and reads. But as a student and later when you begin to practice, you will be expected to recall a surprising amount of information. The better your memory, the easier this will be. For most people, memory is imperfect. Everyone needs reminding from time to time. The best reminders are well-organized, written notes.

The goal of good note taking is to capture key words, ideas, and concepts in short phrases.

Like good study habits, the best note-taking system is the one that works for you. If you already have a note-taking system, use it. If taking notes is not something you normally do, develop a system now. It will be indispensable to you as a student and will continue to work for you after you've graduated.

The advantages of note taking far outweigh getting used to writing them. The main benefit is higher grades. Notes are a written record of what you hear and read. Well-taken, clearly written notes record important facts and ideas that are buried in books and lectures. They tell you what your instructor emphasizes as important, and they reinforce information as you get it. When used properly, they will help you to review and remember what you've covered. They are especially helpful when you need them most—for study and review just before quizzes and tests.

Get into the habit of taking notes. Take them in lectures, when you read, when watching films, videos, and demonstrations, during clinical rounds, and in any other situation where you are being given information to learn and remember.

If note taking does not come naturally to you, or if you have problems keeping good notes, ask your instructor for help immediately. The sooner you begin a set of organized notes, the easier it will be to record, remember, and review the material you're being taught.

There are many kinds of notebooks, and individual preference will determine which you use. Some students prefer keeping all their notes in one loose-leaf notebook with subject dividers. A single notebook keeps and organizes all notes for all classes in one place. Making additions or deletions, or moving pages or sections from one place to another, is simplified. Others like individual notebooks for each subject. An alternative to notebooks is index cards. They allow easy filing and cross-indexing but are less portable and convenient.

For legibility and neatness, use lined paper and write on one side only. The blank facing page can be used for additions or comments to the main notes. Date each set of notes. It's also a good idea to identify each page of notes by course, instructor, or subject, and to number them if they are in loose-leaf form, so that they can be reorganized if they get out of sequence.

When taking notes, sit where you can be comfortable, as close to the lecturer as possible. Make sure you have a clear view of the chalkboard so that you can read your instructor's notes. They should be used as guidelines to organize your own notes. Sit comfortably. Good posture will help you keep alert.

Missed lectures mean missing notes. If you miss a lecture or class, make arrangements to get notes from a classmate to avoid blanks in your notebook and to keep up with the course. Tape-recording a lecture can be helpful if you miss one, but regularly taping lectures wastes time, just as word-for-word notes do.

Note taking is easier when reading assignments are kept up-to-date, because the information in one reinforces the other. A good general rule is to have your reading assignment done before a lecture and, if possible, to review it briefly so that you will be prepared to take notes on new information.

Guidelines for Taking Clear Notes

1. *Listen.* Pay attention to what is being said; avoid distractions; watch, as well as listen to, the speaker.
2. *List.* Write down the main ideas, facts, and supporting data; write down the speaker's chalkboard notes; write down your questions if something is not clear.
3. *Read.* Read your notes as soon as possible after taking them; fill in with any material you remember but didn't write down.
4. *Review.* Review your notes on the day they were made, just before the next lecture in that subject, and before exams.

When listening to a lecture, keep your ears tuned for key words and phrases. Listen and watch for signals from your instructor that indicate what is considered to be important. Phrases such as "will be on the exam," "studies have shown," "the main reason for," "the important thing to remember," and similar remarks are strong suggestions that what will be said next should be written down.

Also, if your instructor pauses, repeats information, slows down the delivery of information, or underlines anything on the board, you can assume it's important. If you pay attention, after a few lectures you'll learn the instructor's style and will know when to write and when to listen.

Be sure to record the notes, diagrams, charts, dates, and other data your instructor writes on the chalkboard.

Your writing style should be what is most comfortable for you. But information may come faster than you can keep up with while using normal writing. If you know shorthand or can improvise a personal shorthand to condense what you hear, you will be able to devote your attention to the lecture. Use underlines for emphasis. Number lists. Eliminate vowels in words to shorten them. Leave out unnecessary words. Shorten sentences.

The standard abbreviations and terms used in charting that you'll be learning can double as shorthand in your note taking. A complete list can be found in Appendix A.

Be cautious when taking abbreviated notes. Although it is easy to abbreviate words, it is sometimes difficult to recall what your abbreviation means. This is especially true when you are building a medical and nursing vocabulary. Completely write or print words that are new to you. If you decide to abbreviate, write the abbreviation in parentheses next to the word. You can use the abbreviation for the new word from that point on, because you have a record of what a particular abbreviation means to you.

Avoid doodling on your note pages and letting your concentration wander. Concentrate on what is being said and condense what you hear into brief, legible notes.

An example of notes from a nursing lecture might read like this:

Warm Soaks

1. Normal saline solution (NSS)
2. Temp 105-110 degrees Fahrenheit (F)
3. 3 times a day (t.i.d.)
4. 20 min.

The next time the lecturer refers to normal saline solution, you need only write "NSS" in your notes; when reference is made to three times a day, you need only write "t.i.d.," and so forth.

Studying

Studying is the process of attentively applying the mind to learn or understand a topic or subject. How much time you have to study will be clear from your schedule. The choice of how to study is up to you.

Study habits are learning tools. Good study habits combined with a desire to learn are essential to success as a student. Both are under your control.

If you have study habits that worked in the past with good results, use them. If your study skills are rusty or you don't have a study method, use these guidelines:

Study Suggestions

1. Set regular times for study and mark them in your schedule.
2. Establish routine places with minimum distractions to study.
3. Set aside a minimum of study time for each hour spent in class.
4. Allow enough time to study each subject.
5. Schedule your study time by priorities.
6. Study the most important subjects first.
7. Study hard subjects before easy subjects.
8. Set the time you'll need for each subject by the difficulty of the material.

9. Revise your schedule and priorities according to need.
10. Take short rests every 45 to 60 minutes of study time.
11. Study just before and right after classes.
12. Study when your energy level is up.
13. Have all necessary books, papers, notes, and other study material on hand before starting.
14. Study dissimilar subjects in each session to keep you and the material fresh.
15. Avoid distractions and interruptions and deal with them quickly when they occur.
16. Take advantage of instructor review sessions and student study groups

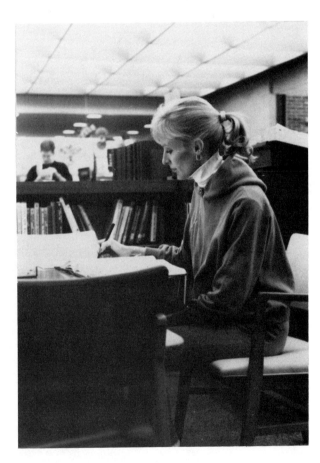

Good study habits will help you succeed. (Photograph courtesy of Laurie Cooper.)

In general, shorter sessions are less tiring than long ones and allow better concentration. Limiting the length of each session makes them more productive.

Proper rest and nutrition are important to clear thinking. Be as comfortable as possible, but avoid conditions that make you drowsy.

Where you study can be as important as how you study. Choose places where the lighting is good, the temperature is comfortable and noise and the opportunity for distraction are at a minimum. And always resist the temptation to give in to anything that interferes with scheduled study time.

Once you establish a study pattern, stick with it. There will be times when you will have to make adjustments. Handle them as they come along and return to your normal pattern when they're done.

Your study schedule should be a part of your life, not all of it. Allow yourself some free time to do the things you enjoy.

The better organized you are, the easier your life as a student nurse will be. This is especially true if school and study do not come easily for you. If getting organized is difficult, ask your adviser, an instructor, or another student who has these skills for help.

Computer-Assisted Instruction

Computers are a growing part of nursing. They are used routinely for data and record keeping, information retrieval, diagnostic and therapeutic procedures, and inventory control.

It is likely you will use computers at some time in your nursing career. You already may have computer experience. Your program may have a computer course component or use them in instruction.

The sooner you familiarize yourself with computers and what they do, the easier it will be to use them. Take advantage of any opportunity to learn and use them. They can help you with your studies now, and knowing how to use them can be an asset to you when you begin practice.

Using a computer does not require any special skills beyond the ability to read. Basically, computer programs, which are instructions to do a task, display written information on a screen. A computer-assisted teaching program, for example, presents information to be learned in short bits, one or a few pieces at a time. The information is repeated a short time later to reinforce the learning. Computer programs show the user what to do step by step. Ask your instructor for help if you have problems.

Audiovisual Instruction

Audiovisual (A/V) instruction, through cable television, video cassettes, films, filmstrips, and other visual media, extends your classroom to places and people you might otherwise only hear or read about. Clinical demonstrations, nursing procedures, and your own performance in skills and techniques can be reviewed conveniently and as often as desired on video tapes.

Treat A/V presentations with the same approach as lectures. Record the information in your notes just as you do in a lecture.

Assignments

Most days you'll be given reading or written assignments to do outside of class. They are an important part of your program. They are intended to introduce new material or reinforce material already covered. A few simple guidelines will help you to do them.

Reading Assignments

Good reading skills are the foundation of successful studying. Reading is easier if one is mentally and physically prepared. Review the guidelines for study on page 11, because studying and reading go hand in hand. In addition:

1. Read in a quiet place with a minimum of interruption or distraction.
2. Adjust temperature and lighting to a comfortable level.
3. Sit upright in a comfortable chair.
4. Avoid reading on a full or empty stomach.
5. Hold your book at a comfortable angle.

To help you to concentrate on what you are reading, to increase your reading speed, and to improve your ability to recall what you read, a popular shortcut called the SQ3R (survey-question-read-recite-review) method will be useful if you don't have a reading system of your own. Use it as follows:

Survey the title, chapter heads, table of contents, preface, introduction, first and last paragraphs, italicized passages, graphs, illustrations, photos, and questions at the end before you begin normal reading.

Question what you will be reading. Think about it before you begin.

Read by skimming first to find and look up unknown words. Then read for content. Take notes as you read. Summarize them after you have finished.

Recite aloud or silently the substance of what you've read. Repeat it as often as you have to, to get the material firmly fixed in your mind.

Review the material before going on to the next task.

Written Assignments

Written assignments, usually in the form of term papers, case studies, and care plans, are a part of your education. You may be given a topic or be asked to choose one. Once you have a topic, the following five steps will help to get you through most papers.

1. Collect the material—books, notes, papers, articles, and other reference matter—your paper is to be based on. The amount of reference material you need will be determined by the assigned length of the paper.
2. Organize and then outline the reference material. A sample outline for a short paper follows:
   I. **Introduction** (states purpose of paper)
      Say what you're going to say. Open with a topic sentence and follow with a short background or history.
   II. **Body** (states main ideas and details)
      Develop the paper's purpose, using research material to substantiate your case. State the main idea and then give details for each main idea you are presenting.
   III. **Conclusion** (states what was said)
      Briefly summarize what you've said in the paper.
3. Write your first draft from beginning to end. Avoid rewriting and editing the first time through.
4. Read your first draft, add notes, make changes and revisions, and then write the final draft.
5. Proofread your final draft and make corrections before handing the paper in.

Reference Material

Books and Other Materials

Beyond lectures, the main source for the information you will need is found in books and other printed material. Except for textbooks and others you own, you will use library books. Knowing which books to read and how to use a library to find them are basic tools for every student. Time spent familiarizing yourself with nursing books and how to use a library now will save you hours of work throughout your program and career.

Most of the books you will use will be recommended by your instructors and other authorities. Trust their judgment. They speak from experience.

A variety of reference material is available. It includes books, journals, magazines, pamphlets, and audiovisual items. General reference books are dictionaries and encyclopedias.

Textbooks, reference books, and most other nonfiction books containing information are organized to simplify finding the information. A table of contents at the front of a book lists each chapter by title, often with a brief description of the topic covered in that chapter. Page numbers indicate where to find the specific chapter.

An index will be found at the back of most books. The index lists specific items in alphabetical order. Names, subjects, and individual topic-related words are in a good index. If you want to find where in the book to look for "psychologists," for example, look under *P.* The word "psychologist" will be listed, followed by the page or pages where it is used.

Use tables of contents and indexes to quickly obtain the information you need.

Appendixes (appendices) are separate sections of related material found at the back of books. A book may have an appendix in which the addresses of nursing organizations are listed, for example. Reference to an appendix is usually made in the body of the book. An item will be followed by a note in this form: See Appendix A, Common Medical Abbreviations.

Glossaries are separate sections listing vocabulary words special to the topic of the book, such as a glossary of nursing terms.

Textbooks and other technical material will be your primary sources for information. However, health-oriented books and magazines and popular consumer magazine articles frequently present good, readable, general health information that can be used to supplement your other reading. Follow your instructor's advice regarding nontechnical sources.

Choose wisely when buying books other than those your course requires. Nursing books are revised often to keep up with change.

Official journals of nursing and other health care organizations provide the latest news and information long before it can be published in books. Your program, library, or instructors may have copies of journals available. You may wish to buy your own subscriptions, but it is a good idea to become acquainted with the various journals first to ensure buying those which fit your needs.

When buying reference material of any kind on your own, see that it's up-to-date, accurate, and reliable. Your instructor is the authority.

Using Libraries

Your program may have its own library or may provide access to one at a nearby hospital or other health care facility. Public libraries, especially central libraries in larger cities, will also have nursing and medical reference material.

Using a library is not difficult. It requires familiarity with how to use a card catalogue and with the location of books. The process is systematized so that every library is organized in the same basic way.

The card catalogue consists of two alphabetical files of 3- by 5-inch cards. One file lists books by author's name. The other file lists books by subject. The author card file has a card for each author whose books are kept in the library. The card lists each of the author's books. Each book is identified by a catalogue number. The catalogue number corresponds to the number written on the book itself. Books are organized on the shelves according to their catalogue number. The plan of organization—where to find the book you are seeking—will be found near the card catalogue.

The subject card file lists books by subject. For example, you will find nursing books in the drawer labeled "N." An index card in the drawer will say "Nursing." Behind it will be a card for each book in the library that pertains to nursing. The book's author, catalogue number, and other information is listed. Use the catalogue number to locate the book on the shelves.

If you have difficulty finding the book or reference material you need, ask the librarian for help. He will be more than willing to assist you.

Taking Tests

Tests are a fact of life for students. Getting through them will be easier if you are prepared. The energy that tests stimulate can be used to your advantage. Direct the energy to preparing for the test, rather than wasting it in unproductive nervous activity.

Preparation for tests includes planned study and review sessions. Be sure of the exact location and the time the test will be given. Know the kind of test it will be (for example, true/false, essay, multiple choice) and the subject or subjects it will cover.

A general strategy for test taking includes the following:

1. Before the exam begins, make sure you understand the directions and what you're supposed to do. If you're uncertain, ask questions before you begin.
2. Look over the whole exam before you begin to answer questions to estimate how much time each section will take. Make a note of your estimate so that you can gauge your progress once you are under way.
3. Be certain you understand the relative grading weights of different sections. Some parts of a test may count more than others. Use this information to determine where to spend more or less time.

   4. Differentiate between hard and easy sections or questions.
   5. Once you have done steps 2, 3, and 4, make a test-taking plan based on your evaluation and stick to it. For example, you can go straight through the test, or do either the hard or easy material first.
   6. When you have a plan, proceed with the test. Pay just enough attention to the time to keep to your plan.

Some test-taking hints are as follows:

On Mixed Easy to Hard Questions

- Do easy questions first to build confidence.
- Mark hard questions with an *x* and harder ones with *xx*, and answer them in order as time allows.
- "Hard" and "easy" are determined by what you know.

On Multiple-Choice Tests

- Find out before the test if you will be penalized for guessing.
- When guessing, trust your first response as correct.
- Eliminate two or more answers before guessing.
- Use what you learn from one question to help answer others.
- Answers with "all," "never," and "always" are generally incorrect.

On Essay Questions

- Think through each answer before writing.
- Make a brief outline.
- Allot an appropriate amount of time for each answer.
- Answer the easy questions first.
- If time is short, get important information down first.

After completing an exam, use any remaining time to review your answers.

Standardized Examinations

Classroom exams are designed to test your knowledge of specific subjects learned over a limited time. Standardized tests show how much of a range of subjects you've learned through all or a portion of your education. They compare your knowledge with students around the country. The comparisons are usually given in percentile rankings. An evaluation of your potential can be based on the comparison.

   No real method of preparation for taking standardized exams is possible because they draw on a broad range of material learned over a long time. However, before taking a standardized test, you may find it helpful to review a similar test to familiarize yourself with the format and types of questions asked. Also, reviewing material that is to be covered in a standardized test will help you remember what you have already learned.

When taking a standardized test, be sure you understand the directions and follow them. Don't make any extra marks on the answer sheet, and be certain to mark the boxes that go with the questions. If you get out of sequence, every answer will be wrong.

Standardized tests may penalize you for guessing. The test directions or the person administering the test will tell you. If you are uncertain, ask.

Read all the answers before marking one, and answer only those you're sure of first. Review skipped answers after you're finished.

If the test doesn't penalize for guessing, eliminate the answers you know are wrong and guess from those remaining.

Clinical Instruction

Clinical instruction is arranged by the faculty to give you practical experience in the care of patients in the health care setting. Your first clinical assignment might be in a nursing home or in a hospital. Regardless of where you are assigned, you will be expected to apply what you learned in the classroom to the care of the patient. This will require you to *integrate* everything you learned in class to the care of the particular patient.

Before you begin to care for your patient, you should review your textbooks and notes to be sure you correctly understand the patient's condition, the treatment being given, and the procedures you will be performing. In the beginning, your instructor will help you define what you are permitted to do. As you gain experience and clinical skills, you will be expected to identify those skills you can perform independently and those which require instructor observation.

Most often, your day will start with a short "preconference." During this time your instructor will review the instructional plan for the day. You and your classmates will be given an opportunity to ask questions about your assignments, and your instructor may give specific instructions about new treatments or procedures that you may be expected to complete during your clinical time. It is important that you write these notes on a small notepad that will fit into your pocket. It is easy in the rush of the clinical environment to forget the directions your instructor gave you. It is also easy to forget what you are expected to do for your patients.

The majority of your clinical time will be spent learning to care for patients. Your instructor is usually responsible for your activities in the patient unit, and you must keep him or her informed of any changes in your

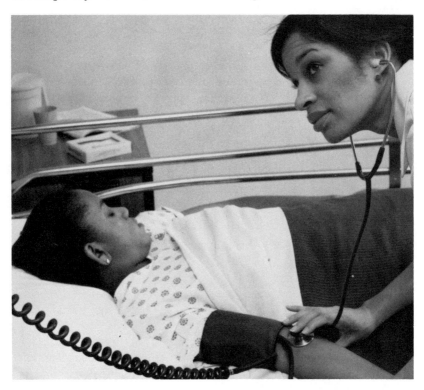

Learning to care for patients is the focus of your clinical experience.

patient's condition. Your instructor will frequently ask you questions about your patient's disease, treatments, family, procedures, and so forth. This is really an oral quiz. You should be prepared to answer these questions at any time.

Meal and break times are assigned by your instructor or the nurse in charge of the unit. Assignments are made to ensure that adequate nursing personnel are always present on the patient unit. It is easy to understand why it is important to plan your activities so that you can leave the unit on time and return on time.

Your clinical day may conclude with a "postconference." A variety of activities usually occur during postconference. Students may present pre-assigned reports to the class, the instructor may discuss the care of a particular patient, a guest speaker may present a topic of special interest, or new equipment or procedures may be demonstrated. Note taking is important. You are responsible for learning the material presented during your clinical day, just as you are for learning the material presented during a classroom lecture.

Attendance during your clinical assignments is crucial to developing nursing skills. Your classmates and the nursing staff depend on you. Being late is disruptive to the care of the patient, to your own organization, to the nursing staff, to your classmates, and to your instructor. Your absence requires that your assignment be given to someone else, often at the last minute. Being on time is an essential personal trait of a nurse.

There are occasions when something unavoidable happens and you must be late or absent. Your instructor will tell you how to handle these situations. You will be expected to comply with your program regulations.

Discussion Questions/Learning Activities

1. What do you think will be the most difficult adjustment you will have to make to attend school? What do you think you will do to make the adjustment?
2. Construct a schedule similar to the schedule shown in Table 1-1 and follow it closely for 1 week. What changes do you think you should make in your schedule and why?
3. Compare your note-taking system with that of some of your classmates. Look for ideas that will help you with your notes.
4. Discuss studying techniques with other students in your class. Which techniques might you be able to use that you had not thought of before?
5. What adjustments could you make in your study schedule to compensate for a short-term personal or family emergency?
6. What are the procedures for using library facilities and how can you get assistance in finding information in your library?
7. Share techniques that you and your classmates use to handle anxiety associated with taking exams.

Suggested Readings

Kesselman-Turkel J, Peterson F: Study Smarts: How to Learn More in Less Time. Chicago, Contemporary Books, 1981.

Kesselman-Turkel J, Peterson F: Test Taking Strategies. Chicago, Contemporary Books, 1981.

Kesselman-Turkel J, Peterson F: Note Taking Made Easy. Chicago, Contemporary Books, 1982.

Kesselman-Turkel J, Peterson F: Getting It Down: How to Put Your Ideas on Paper. Chicago, Contemporary Books, 1983.

Morgan CT: How to Study. New York, McGraw-Hill, 1979.

2 The Student Nurse as a Person

Objectives

When you complete this chapter, you should be able to:

Name the five levels of human needs described by Maslow.

Identify at least six factors that should enhance your personal health.

Describe several personal characteristics that contribute to maintaining good mental health.

Explain the role of socializing and recreation in developing positive physical and mental health.

Describe your personal values and beliefs related to health.

Listen to the views and opinions of others with respect.

Recognize your own physical and mental limits and live within those boundaries.

Linda, an LPN working nights at a nursing home, was summoned to her patient's room by the blinking light over the room door. The corridors were silent. She stepped into the room, which was lighted by the glow of a small lamp. Her patient, Mrs. Mulrooney, was awake. "Can I help you?" Linda asked.

Mrs. Mulrooney nodded. "I'd like a glass of water," she said.

Linda poured a fresh glass and put it to Mrs. Mulrooney's lips. She noticed the old woman was trembling. "Is something wrong?" Linda asked.

Mrs. Mulrooney looked to the side of her bed. "The bedside rails are broken," she whispered.

Linda smiled. "No, Mrs. Mulrooney. They were repaired just today. Remember?"

The old woman looked puzzled. "Was that today?"

Linda put the glass on the night stand. "Yes," she said. "You don't have to worry." She tucked the blanket under her patient's chin.

The old woman smiled and said, I feel safer with the bed rails up. She then touched the nurse's hand. "You make me feel so good," she said.

Linda returned the gesture with a gentle touch. "I'm glad," she said. "You're very important to me."

Mrs. Mulrooney beamed. "I am?" she asked.

Linda stroked her patient's forehead. "Of course you are. You're important to all of us."

For a moment Mrs. Mulrooney said nothing. She was thinking. Then she smiled. "I guess I am," she said proudly. "I should be. I lived a good life. I have two wonderful children and five grandchildren . . ."

Linda stepped to the door as the old woman's eyes began to close in sleep.

"I think I did with my life what I was supposed to," Mrs. Mulrooney said.

"I think so, too," Linda whispered into the room. Mrs. Mulrooney was asleep. Her face was calm. She was smiling.

Human Needs

All people have needs. Because these needs are necessary for survival and health, they are called basic human needs. The story presented above illustrates five categories of human needs identified by Dr. Abraham Maslow, an authority in the field of psychology. They are as follows:

1. Physiological ("I'd like a glass of water.")
2. Safety and security ("I feel safer with the bed rails up.")
3. Love and belonging ("You make me feel so good.")
4. Self-esteem and recognition ("You're very important . . .")
5. Fulfillment ("I think I did with my life what I was supposed to.")

According to Maslow, these five categories of needs can be ordered from simple to complex. Figure 2-1 illustrates Maslow's different levels of human needs. Physical survival and safety come before love and belonging, followed by the need for self-esteem and for fulfillment.

Working with others requires understanding their needs. It also requires understanding your own needs. Unless your needs are recognized, it is difficult to give full attention to the needs of others.

The more you work with people, the more opportunity you will have to learn about yourself. The opportunity begins now. Your self-fulfillment will grow if you know what your needs are and what you must do to satisfy them.

Your Physical Health and Well-Being

Physical health is the absence of disease, pain, or abnormal condition. It is in a constant state of change as the body adapts to conditions and events affecting it. Good physical health is important for anyone in health care.

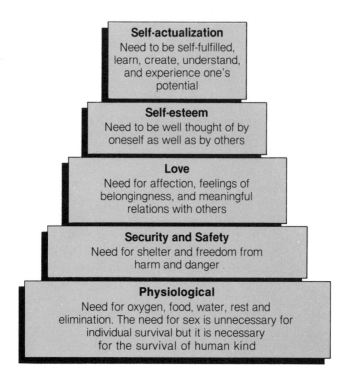

Figure 2-1. Maslow's five levels of human needs.

Good health makes it easier for you to perform your duties. Being healthy is an example you should try to set for your patients. To be healthy, you have to pay attention to your body as though you were your own patient.

When you begin caring for patients, a question you often will ask them will be, "How are you feeling today?" The answers your patients supply will tell you what to do for them.

It isn't necessary to ask yourself this question. You already know the answer. But you do have to respond to what your body tells you. Waiting for a problem to develop is not the best way to ensure good health. Preventing problems, whenever possible, is. Health problems can be minimized through regular physical exams and dental checkups.

Your program may offer health-related services to its students that include exams and checkups. Make use of them. If medical services are provided, you will be expected to pay for them according to established policies. Whenever you have questions regarding charges for your own health care, don't be reluctant to ask about them ahead of time.

If charges for your medical care are reduced as a courtesy by a treating physician, it is a sign of good manners to express your appreciation. On the other hand, it is improper to ask for medical advice for yourself or your family from the physicians you work with while on duty.

Diet

"You are what you eat" is more than a clever saying; it is true. Your daily performance is directly affected by what you eat or don't eat. You'll learn the fundamentals of diet and nutrition. The consequences of poor eating habits versus balanced nutrition are a matter of scientific record. Your own experience tells you that heavy meals produce drowsiness, hunger disrupts concentration, too much caffeine causes jitters, alcohol impairs judgment, and too many calories lead to overweight.

Nurses and others whose work is demanding, often intense, and sometimes awkwardly scheduled, may be open to breaking the rules of good nutrition. Students may also adjust their eating habits to meet the daily requirements of classes, study time, and their personal life, even though both their mental activity and their physical activity demand peak performance. As a student, you will benefit from good eating habits.

Start each day with a balanced breakfast. Eat small, balanced, nourishing meals to maintain energy and stamina through the rest of the day. Avoid snacks with high sugar content. They produce unstable blood sugar levels while adding calories. Whatever your weight, calories that don't help you to study, keep you alert, or ward off exhaustion have no place in your diet. Learn your ideal weight and maintain it. A nurse who is overweight will have difficulty advising patients to diet. If you have to diet, avoid crash diets and diets that exclude variety.

Eat a variety of foods that include some of each of the four food groups recommended by the National Academy of Sciences–National Research Council: (1) dairy, (2) meat, including fish, eggs, and poultry, (3) vegetables and fruit, and (4) bread and cereal. Include adequate fiber in your daily diet and avoid excessive amounts of caffeine, salt, saturated fats and cholesterol, and alcohol.

Rest and Exercise

Studying and clinical experience may create a double drain on your energy because of the demand for both physical activity and mental activity. Having to concentrate while keeping up with a busy schedule may make you more tired more than you're used to. You may require more rest. Watch for signs of fatigue—indifference, sluggishness, personality changes, a drab physical appearance—to prevent the situation from growing worse.

Mental alertness and physical endurance are qualities you must have as a student and throughout your career. They depend in large measure on how well you rest. You can't "save up" on sleep. The amount of sleep needed varies with the individual, so only you will know if you're getting enough. Seven to eight hours a night is average, although some people manage on less and others need more. Experiment to learn your own limits and then stay within them to maintain a consistent level of energy.

Restful deep sleep is better than tense light sleep. How well you sleep is indicated by how rested you feel after you've been up a short time in the morning. How one prepares for sleep is a personal practice, but in general, to ensure quality sleep, relax before going to bed, avoid eating or drinking before retiring, sleep on a firm mattress, and provide comfortable temperature and ventilation.

To increase your endurance during the day, take scheduled rest breaks. It is not necessary to nap, but if you can, let your body and mind enjoy a few moments of peace by reducing or eliminating physical and mental activity.

A scheduled program of specific exercise also helps to keep the body working efficiently. Even though your work may be physically demanding, if parts of your body are neglected, the effect on them is the same as having no exercise at all. Walking, swimming, aerobic workouts, jogging, and bicycling are exercises that use a full range of body activity. To help keep your energy levels high, your body tone good, and your weight in control, engage in a sport or exercise that matches or slightly exceeds your ability. You may find it helpful to join a group of other students or friends in scheduled exercise sessions two or three times a week.

Oral Hygiene and Dental Health

You will be working closely with patients, staff, members, and others who will appreciate your attention to keeping your teeth and breath attractive. A pleasant smile can be an asset. Regular dental checkups will find problems such as cavities, decay, and gum disease, and vigorous daily brushing and periodic freshening will help to ensure a clean, healthy mouth. Consider seeing a dentist or orthodontist if cosmetic treatment is indicated for dentition problems (poor bite), particularly if they affect your self-confidence or the image you'd like to project.

Personal Hygiene

Cleanliness in health services begins with personal hygiene. It affects your image and may affect your susceptibility to cross infection and disease. Your personal care must reflect the higher overall standards expected from people in health care.

Basic personal care includes clean skin, clean, neatly combed or brushed hair, and the absence of body odor. Hands and nails must be clean.

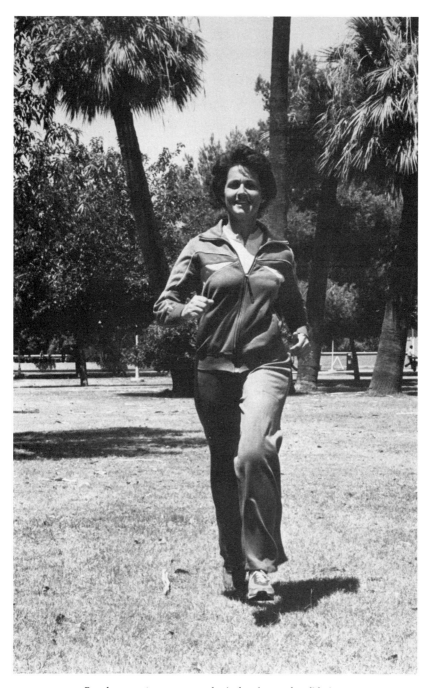

Regular exercise promotes physical and mental well-being.

If the use of makeup and perfume, the length of nails and the use of nail polish, and types of hair styles are covered in policies set by your program and later by your employer, follow them. Perfumes and scented deodorants and hair sprays may create discomfort in patients and can aggravate allergies. If the decision on grooming aids is up to you, a moderate approach is best. If you are unsure, ask someone whose opinion you respect for advice.

Clothing and Uniforms

Your uniform is a symbol of your vocation. It is often the first thing people notice, especially patients, who identify it with their stay in a hospital or health care facility. It makes a statement about you, what you stand for, and your authority. It should be worn only at work.

Maintain a positive impression by wearing uniforms, caps (if required), and other clothing that are clean, pressed, and fresh. Shoes are also a part of your uniform and should be clean and in good repair. They should be comfortable and of a style that is consistent with your work and image.

Pins, name tags, and other devices that identify you, your institution, or your affiliations should be worn in accordance with policies set forth by your employer, your state, or the associations they represent.

Posture

How you stand, sit, walk, and carry your body is a matter of habit by now. If your habits are good, there's no need to change them. On the other hand, if your posture is not good, your appearance, performance, and energy level will improve if you change it—most people's do.

Basic good posture is to hold your body straight. When standing, keep your back straight and your head up. Walk with your shoulders back and your head erect. When sitting, keep your back straight and both feet on the floor. Be relaxed in your posture, not rigid. Keeping muscles tense will tire you quickly.

Body language, which is how you hold and carry yourself, can reflect how you feel physically, some of what you feel about yourself, and some of what you feel about others.

For example, standing straight expresses self-confidence. Slouching reduces your authority. Talking to someone with your arms folded tightly across your chest puts people off. Facing them directly in a straightforward, relaxed manner encourages a positive response.

Smoking

People who smoke give many excuses for their habit, but nobody can claim it is for good health. The public is keenly aware of the negative effects of smoking. Studies clearly show that some heart disease, lung cancer, chronic obstructive pulmonary disease (COPD), and other ailments can be directly linked to smoking. You will learn more about the health dangers that are associated with smoking as your knowledge about health increases. You'll see patients whose only reason for being ill is related to smoking, and some of them, tragically, are terminally ill. Others will have illnesses that smoking complicates by making manageable conditions worse and marginal sickness serious. In the air or on one's clothes, smoke is an irritant. For a patient whose well-being depends on optimum conditions, the smell of smoke, whether first or second hand, is contraindicated.

There is another side to the smoking question for you as a student nurse. As a highly visible member of the health professions, your example to others can affect how they view their own smoking. A health practitioner who smokes gives unspoken approval to the habit.

If you smoke, you have an obligation not to do so when or where it will affect others in any way. For your good health and the health and comfort of those you're around, look closely at your excuses for smoking and its consequences. You'll find plenty of reasons to quit. Groups are available for those who want to quit but have trouble doing so.

Chemical Dependence

The use and abuse of controlled substances, the so-called "hard" and "soft" drugs—such as heroin, cocaine, amphetamines, barbiturates, Quaaludes, hashish, and marijuana—and alcohol have increased greatly in the United States and around the world over the past 20 years. It is a growing, serious problem. The "recreational" use of drugs and alcohol—weekend and occasional use—remains high. More people are using controlled substances during the week, both on and off the job.

Addiction—uncontrollable, compulsive dependence—and *habituation*—psychological and emotional dependence without addiction—often result from continued use of drugs and alcohol. Both forms of dependence affect every socioeconomic group. The degree of dependence can vary widely among individuals.

Recent studies suggest that some people are more likely to develop an addiction than others, but there are no simple ways to determine who they are. Don't be lulled into thinking that the use of drugs is harmless, either for yourself or people you know. Being well informed about drug and alcohol use is your best defense against abuse.

The illegal use or possession of controlled drugs can be used to deny, suspend, or revoke your license—or prevent you from taking the licensure exam at all. Your school and the clinical facilities used in your program are certain to have policies on drug use.

The first-hand knowledge of the effects of drugs and alcohol you gain through your program should be a constant reminder to you to protect your health and career. Others who are not so fortunate may approach you because of your professional association with the use of drugs in a hospital or institution. Make it very clear to them that you neither use, approve of, nor can supply or administer any drugs for any reason unless prescribed by a physician for your patients.

Alcohol is also a drug. It is responsible for more addiction than any other in the United States. Alcoholism, the name given to alcohol addiction, is a major health problem and an economic drain. It's the direct cause of enormous suffering and expense from liver and kidney disease, psychological disturbances, crippling injury, illness, family disruption, and death.

There is a high rate of drug and alcohol abuse among nurses. Their dependence is doubly tragic because it affects not only their own lives, families, and careers, but the lives of their patients as well.

Whatever your personal beliefs and feelings about the use of alcohol and drugs, there is never justification for using these substances at work or for abusing them at any other time. Your education and the experiences you will have will demonstrate the disastrous effects of drug and alcohol abuse on people's lives and health. The likelihood of serious disciplinary action in your program or by an employer in the future—many use prehiring drug screenings—is ample reason for you to avoid their use and abuse.

As a nurse, your relationship with drug and alcohol use is twofold. You must be very cautious of it in your own life, and you must also empathize with your patients who have a problem.

Personal Illness and Your Patients

The same standards of care and protection you use when working with patients with transmissible illness apply to you when you are ill. The difference is that although you may be informed about your patients' health, they know nothing of yours.

It is your obligation to avoid contaminating a patient or his environment when you have any illness that could harm or affect a patient's health or well-being. This applies to transmissible diseases, from common colds to serious infections, and to conditions that have a negative psychological effect, such as coughs, rashes, and other symptoms of disease.

Your program or clinical facility policies may be explicit on matters of personal illness. If not, your good judgment will tell you when to avoid exposing co-workers and patients if you are ill. Your awareness of the state of your health is your best guide to protecting yourself and others.

Sexually Transmitted Diseases

The emergence of acquired immune deficiency syndrome (AIDS) has greatly increased public awareness of sexually transmitted diseases (STDs), but there is still a lot of misinformation and fear about them. Providing health information to others is a service performed by nurses. As a student nurse, you may be asked questions about STDs. Your ability to answer them will increase as your education progresses.

There are many sexually transmitted diseases. Once called veneral diseases, they include syphilis, gonorrhea, herpes, and others. Their complications can be serious and may lead to death. Those which are not directly life threatening can lead to infections and illnesses that are. Many STDs can lead to sterility and other reproductive problems.

Although some STDs can be transmitted by blood transfusion and other means, they are generally associated with human sexuality, a subject that many find difficult to talk about. Your willingness to be open, frank, and honest about STDs is important to patients and others who seek information, because the best method to control these diseases is through education. As a student nurse, what you have to say is valuable.

You should not make judgments that will keep information about STDs from those who need it. STDs can be acquired by anyone who is sexually active, and there are no social, economic, racial, or other barriers. Because STDs always involve two or more people, the sex partners of anyone with a sexually transmitted disease should be informed so that they can seek medical attention. Also, because reinfection of a partner is likely if only one is treated, all partners must get treatment to contain the chain of infection.

Learn accurate, scientific information about what causes STDs, what their incubation periods are, how they are transmitted, how to identify them, and what to do to prevent and treat them. Armed with this information, you can do much to promote good health for yourself and others. For further information on sexually transmitted diseases, refer to Appendix B.

Your Emotional Health

Good emotional health is the overall contentment, satisfaction, and peace of mind that comes from a life that is minimally disturbed by complications of family, school, work, and community. In brief, it hinges on the ability to cope. Emotional health goes beyond mental illness and applies not only to patients but to everyone.

Everyone experiences upsets in life. It is not the degree of upset but how it is handled that determines the state of one's mental health. There is no point on a scale or single characteristic that separates someone who is mentally healthy from one who is mentally ill.

Almost everyone has personality quirks that are managed appropriately and can't be considered true disorders. On the other hand, as many as 1 out of 10 Americans need professional help for mental disorders, whether they seek it or not. How much you are in charge of your own mental well-being is an indication of maturity and will influence your success in life and work.

Mature students are those who see a need to act and then act responsibly. They will act independently if the duty is clearly theirs or willingly under the direction of others when asked. If uncertain, they are willing to ask questions and request help when needed. They deal with problems as they are, not as they wish they were. When confronted by an unfamiliar task, they know not to attempt it without consulting their instructor or a superior.

Maturity is also the ability to accept constructive criticism. Students who use correction and comment to improve themselves and their work do not personalize the criticism but recognize it as a part of the education they have paid for and expect.

Having personal and vocational maturity also means that nurses should keep an open, analytical mind. They should see the positive side in situations and people that others may not see and work to promote it. They should be open, caring, and friendly, and they should respect their peers, superiors, and other members of their health and administrative team.

Because nurses have the responsibility for people whose attention is fully on themselves, they have to be more understanding than someone without that responsibility.

To meet the emotional demands of nursing, you as a student nurse must begin to develop a good understanding of yourself.

Understanding Yourself

One gains or develops maturity and good mental health through self-understanding. A willingness to look at yourself and your life objectively—self-evaluation—and squarely face what you find will influence how well you succeed.

All of life's experiences, whether good or bad, affect how one sees oneself and provide the opportunity for self-understanding and self-improvement. For example, adapting to divorce can lead to better self-understanding, just as adjusting to being married can. Raising a child alone can provide valuable lessons for living, just as sharing the responsibility with a spouse can. When you evaluate yourself, look at every side and use what you see to build yourself up, rather than tear yourself down.

Without self-understanding, you cannot reasonably expect to understand others and therefore to help them. You are not expected to be fault free; nobody is. But your obligation as a nurse is to care for others. To do that you have to make the effort to limit your self-concerns during your workday so that they don't prevent you from attending to the needs of your patients.

Self-awareness is a lifelong process that produces rewards from the beginning. How deeply you probe is a matter for you to decide. To start, ask yourself how well you really know yourself. Does what you know agree with how others see you? Are you willing to make changes?

Personality

Personality is the collection of behavior and attitudes that sets one person apart from everyone else. You were not born with your personality. You developed it gradually—consciously and unconsciously—as a way of adapting to the circumstances of your life and environment. Personality is not character. Character relates to the conscious, consistent way one reacts to ethical and moral customs and the standards of society.

It is easier to change personality traits than character traits, but neither is altogether easy. It is your personality that interacts with others. Your personality is where to look for traits that need refining, changing, or elimination.

As a nurse, how well you interact with others is important. The personal nature of your work requires you to do more than just get along. You also must inspire positive relationships. Supervisors will expect you to work with minimum supervision. Peers and associates will expect you to do your share of what needs to be done. Your patients will expect you to see to their physical and emotional needs without being asked. To relate positively takes conscious effort, especially in a health care setting, where there is a broad mix of age, culture, and background. Your personality will not work on "automatic pilot" in such a diverse population. You have to be willing to adapt your behavior as new situations occur.

Changing personality traits, especially those that are deep-seated, takes time, but they can be changed if you know what they are. Study yourself as though you were someone else. Make notes of traits you think are positive and those you think detract from a healthy personality. Look among the people you respect for traits that make them stand out, and use them as models. You don't have to adopt them entirely—just use the parts that suit you.

Get input about how others see you from people whose opinions you respect. Make it clear how important their insight is and that you are not looking for flattery. Be willing to accept what they tell you whether you agree with it or not. Use what you learn to change the parts of your personality that would hinder you from becoming a better person and a better nurse.

Personal Values and Beliefs

As individuals, we behave independently, but much of our behavior is a result of learned social customs. When most members of a group express similar behavior, the behavior is called ethnic.

Culture is the sum of ideas, customs, skills, and arts of given groups of people during specified periods. It is the pattern of overall behavior of families, races, nations, or societies and is passed from generation to generation.

Ethnic differences are cultural characteristics that are shared by subgroups within populations. Ethnic groups are identified by customs, language, common history, and other characteristics. An example of a cultural custom is the institution of marriage. The way a given cultural group celebrates weddings is an ethnic difference.

Many people spend much of their lives in the comfort of their own ethnic or cultural heritage, with people with whom they share deep-seated similarities. However, as a consequence of work, some people come into contact with people from widely differing backgrounds.

Because of the nature of nursing, nurses are confronted with a full range of people who differ in age, sex, race, religion, ethnicity, economic status, and other categories. Everyone ages. Everyone is susceptible to illness. Anyone can have an accident. At some time or another, everyone needs health care, even those who don't seek it. When they do, you will be there as a part of the nursing care team to provide it, regardless of who the person is. That's the commitment you are making to nursing.

How you handle patient differences will be a measure of your compassion, understanding, and maturity. It will also depend on your willingness to accept their differences regardless of your personal opinion.

The foundation of your service to your patients is the acknowledgment that their basic needs are the same as everyone else's, including your own.

Your patients experience hunger, but their choice in food may differ from yours. They need clothing, but the style they wear may not be found in your wardrobe. They need shelter, although they may not be your neighbors. They need human kindness, but they may be strangers to you. Everything about your patients may be a "world" away from your own, but when all their cultural and ethnic differences are removed, you are their nurse, they are your patients, and you live in the same world.

Because there are many differences among people, there is a tendency, which comes from the need to survive, to reject another's differences in favor of one's own preferences. This is called prejudice.

Prejudice

Prejudice means prejudgment—forming an opinion about people or things without ample reason or information.

Prejudice is not somethig one is born with. It is behavior that is learned from others, usually early in life. It comes easily because it takes no work or investigation of facts. It only needs one's willingness to go along with someone else's decision, which itself has most likely been accepted from an even more remote source. The result is widely accepted misinformation and misunderstanding that is so durable that virtually nothing can change it.

Everyone has some prejudice and to varying degrees. People who feel good about themselves are less likely to harbor significant prejudices than do people with low self-esteem. People with a poor self-image often redirect their negative feelings about themselves toward others.

Because everyone has prejudices, you must identify your own and work to get rid of them. Left where they are, they will hinder your ability to care for your patients, will get in the way of your career, and will inhibit your personal growth.

Getting rid of prejudices takes courage because it requires you to let go of a part of your self. Old, familiar, comfortable attitudes that you have had from childhood were not all caused consciously or with an intent to hurt anyone. They are usually there because of misinformation, fear, and insecurity.

Stand in front of a mirror and ask yourself, "How many reasons are there for someone who has never met me and does not know me to distrust me, not like me, reject me, or hate me?" The answer is none. It is the same number of reasons anyone can have for prejudging anyone else.

Coping With Stress

Stress is a condition of tension between two opposite forces. The forces can be physical, psychological, economic, or social, alone or in combination. A simple yet descriptive example of physical stress is a hot air balloon tied to the ground by a rope. The balloon wants to rise. The rope wants to hold it down. Tension between the force to rise and the force holding the balloon down makes the rope stretch. If a rope could feel pain, it would hurt. If the rope is not strong enough, it will break. Once the balloon is released, whether by a broken rope or just letting it go, the tension vanishes.

So many situations in life are similar to this analogy that stress has become a word in everyone's vocabulary. A child who wants to go outside but is stopped by a parent because the weather is wet and cold experiences stress. A student facing an important exam experiences stress. A stomach that is overfilled with a holiday meal produces stress. A couple having an argument undergo stress.

Not all stress is harmful. Limited stress before an exam can raise energy levels, for example. But too much stress may result in anxiety, physical illness, psychological distress, fatigue, and other emotional and physical responses. Stress—opposing forces—seeks a response. The nature of the response—how one copes—determines whether the stress is relieved or worsened.

The connection between the mind and body is underscored by stress. A stressful situation always produces a reaction in the body. If the reaction is too great, the odds increase that something will hurt or break. Tension headaches are stress related. So are some ulcers. Nervousness and anxiety result from stress. It is to anyone's advantage to control stress.

The most effective way to control stress is to release the tension before it gets out of hand. Periods of rest will reduce fatigue. A light snack will reduce hunger. Telling someone what is bothering you relieves psychological tension. Confronting a personal fear reduces anxiety.

Managing stress—your own or your patients'—can be accomplished by a number of techniques that combine physical and mental relaxation. In principle, they cause the mind and body to slow down for a brief period or quietly force a change of attention. A progressive relaxation technique, for example, uses a 15- to 30-minute process in which one's attention is put on every part of the body, one part at a time, while one is consciously thinking and feeling relaxation. Another technique, called guided imagery, is one in which the person who wishes to relax uses the imagination to think himself into a pleasant situation, such as lying in the warm sun on a sandy beach. Deep breathing exercises are a part of most stress management techniques.

You can practice stress management techniques on your own or in groups. Group sessions are helpful because they let you share an experience with others, which itself reduces tension. As an individual, you can use simple breathing exercises, such as taking a few deep breaths before an exam or when facing a stressful situation, without elaborate preparation or the need for a quiet, private place.

Stress that gets out of hand can be harmful. When anxiety or other stress-related conditions begin to dominate your life and your efforts to manage stress by yourself are not working, look to others for help. Talking to a friend may be enough. A chat with your instructor may help. Professional counseling is always a good idea when the stress in one's life exceeds the ability to cope. Make use of it.

Some stress management techniques are provided in Appendix C. You may find these suggestions useful for yourself and your patients.

Communication

Communication is the exchange of information between a source and a receiver. It is an important part of nursing, from education to delivery of services.

An example of communication that shows the flow of information (messages) from a source to a receiver is a radio station that is broadcasting a program to listeners. The radio station is the source, the program is the message, and the listener is the receiver.

One-way communication is when the message goes from the source to the receiver and stops, in the way a news program broadcasts information to its listeners.

Two-way communication is when the message from the source encourages the receiver to respond. This can be likened to a radio talk show, in which the host asks listeners to call in with opinions on what they've just heard.

In your program, an example of one-way communication is what occurs in class when your instructor delivers information to you in a lecture.

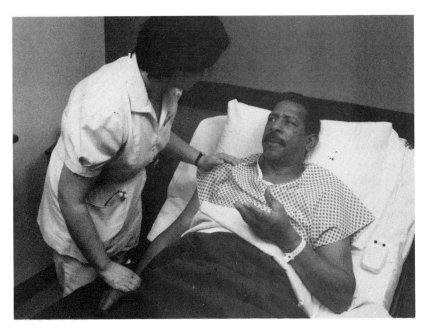

The nurse uses touch to communicate caring.

Two-way communication occurs when your instructor expects you to respond with questions and answers relating to the lecture.

Understanding both kinds of communications and how to use them effectively is fundamental to nursing practice.

Communication can be verbal, nonverbal, or a combination of both.

Verbal communication is language that is most often expressed in speaking and sometimes in writing.

Nonverbal communication is body language, which includes silence, facial expression, and any other actions that do not use words. Examples of nonverbal communication are averting or shaking your head when speaking or being spoken to, impatiently tapping a foot, frowning, yawning, and other expressions that consciously or unconsciously reveal what is really on your mind.

Verbal and nonverbal communication are often used together, but either can be effective without the other.

All five senses are used in communication. In nursing practice, one of the senses, touch, is especially important. Not touching someone can be as cold as silence, just as rough handling can be the physical equivalent of shouting.

Good communication skills are absolutely necessary in nursing because *how* you communicate affects *what* you communicate, and both will influence your relationships with peers, supervisors, and patients. These skills include using correct grammar and vocabulary, speaking clearly in a pleasant voice, using good judgment in what you say, giving simple, straightforward answers to questions, expressing self-confidence, being a good listener without interrupting, using accurate descriptions, and using words and phrases that are appropriate to the listener.

Speaking

How you speak can be as important as what you say, because the sound of your voice and the style of your delivery can communicate hints of hidden meaning, just as body language does. Important messages lose their impact when delivered in a wishy-washy way, and annoying characteristics of speech, such as whining, shouting, or slurring words, detract from what is being said.

Self-consciousness is a big obstacle to clear speaking. If you are uncomfortable when talking, now is the time to analyze your speech habits. Learn which habits are reducing your effectiveness as a speaker and replace them with new ones. Practice your new habits alone at first and then with a friend or classmate. When you begin to feel secure, try them out on strangers. Clear speaking is a skill that can be learned, just as poor speech habits can be unlearned. In a vocation where you will be "on stage" when you work, the sooner you perfect your technique, the easier your work will be.

To improve your spoken verbal communication skills, study the way that you speak. For example, you can use a tape recorder to hear how you sound to others, and speaking in front of a mirror will show you how you look when talking.

When speaking, face the person you're addressing. Keep eye contact and state your words clearly, without skipping syllables or slurring their pronunciation. Use words that you are comfortable with to avoid using terms that sound out of place, even though you understand their meaning. Your words, tone, rhythm, inflection, and posture should work together when you communicate. The failure of any one aspect of communication will detract from what you are saying and may create a wrong impression.

In general, to improve the quality of what you say so that you can be understood easily:

- Organize your thoughts before speaking.
- Avoid set speeches that sound memorized.
- Keep your listener in mind when you're speaking.
- Keep your opinions and values out of communications where they don't belong.
- Use proper technical terms when speaking with colleagues.
- Give complete explanations in plain English when giving technical information to patients and families. (Plain English for technical explanations lets you give comforting answers to questions without wasting time.)
- Restate or repeat in your own words questions or statements by others to make sure you understand what they've said.
- Ask your listener for an opinion or other response. (This lets patients express feelings and fears in a nonthreatening environment.)
- Address people appropriately, as Mr., Mrs., Miss or Ms., according to their wishes.
- Avoid trite terms of endearment, such as honey, dear, or Grandpa, when addressing patients and families.
- Avoid teasing, even if your intention is to raise spirits. (It does not always work and can backfire.)
- Never be sarcastic.
- Avoid giving false reassurances to anyone about your patient's condition. (However well intended, they may be counterproductive.)
- Keep personal opinions out of communications where they don't belong.
- Do your best to sound cheerful even when you don't feel it.

You're not expected to be a professional lecturer, but improving your speech skills will help you make a positive impression.

Listening

Listening is the tool used to receive what another person is communicating. It facilitates the exchange of information. Good listening often comes before observation. You will frequently hear or be told something before seeing it at first hand. For example, you will read a patient's chart or will be told about the patient before meeting him in person.

How good a listener you are affects communication between you and others. It can also influence how well you do your work. By listening closely, you will hear the information being communicated to you. When you are given directions to do something, for example, knowing exactly what a supervisor is telling you will let you work with confidence.

A good listener also gains the confidence of the speaker. Where supervisors are concerned, this translates into approval of you and your performance. Establishing confidence with patients makes working with them easier and, as important, is therapeutic for them as well.

Listening and hearing are not the same. Hearing means only that sound has reached the ears. Listening gives meaning to the sound through conscious attention. Hearing can be tuned out by not paying attention to the sound reaching the ears, whether it's music, someone talking, or the hum of a refrigerator in the background. A mother will be awakened by her baby's soft crying when someone else would not hear it at all.

Good listening habits do not come naturally for everyone, but they can be learned. In conversation or at other times when listening is important, most people focus their attention on what they themselves are saying or thinking, and not on the speaker. This normal egocentricity (focus on the self) conflicts with the need for nurses to be exceptional listeners. There are two steps to good listening:

1. Focus your attention on the speaker to hear what is said
2. Interpret what is said to understand what to do

There's more to being a good listener than clear communication. As an important person in your patients' lives, you will be someone they will turn to express their hopes, fears, opinions, and personal matters. By listening closely to what they say, you will provide an outlet for feelings that they might otherwise keep bottled up. This can help to relieve their stress, which is often a component of illness. And by listening between the lines, you will hear what they really need or want to say.

Being a good listener does not mean to insert yourself or your opinions into your patient's life the way one does in daily social conversation. It also does not mean you have the right to pry. Accept what they tell you without judging what they say. Treat it with total confidentiality. Remember that you are not the patient's only audience but only one of many people in his life at the moment. You should be receptive and open, but it is not your role to be an adviser.

Sharing experiences is a normal part of ordinary conversation, but a patient who relates a significant event in his life is not looking for a similar story from you, and you should not offer any. Nod, smile, and acknowledge that you are listening. Be there for your patients without interrupting. Ask questions as a way to show your interest, but don't ask questions that don't relate to what has been said or questions that can be construed as prying. Don't let boredom or lack of interest show. Be a good, courteous, interested but neutral listener.

Writing

Writing is also verbal communication. Writing something down may be less threatening to you than facing someone and telling him directly, but writing requires the same attention as speaking.

You are already learning the importance of good writing from your note taking. Clear, legible notes release their information whenever it is needed without having to dig it out. Muddled, scribbled, and erratic notes take more time and work to translate than rereading the original material they were taken from.

The need to write clearly does not end when you leave your program. Your ability to write well will be more important to you than ever when you enter practice. Once you begin to record on patients' charts, fill out forms and applications, write requisitions, and do the other writing your daily work will require, how well it is done will have a bearing on your patients' well-being, health, and life.

Neatness, legibility, and precise meaning in as few words as possible are the basics of good writing.

Charting is a special kind of writing skill that has a direct bearing on patient care. Long, vague, or meaningless written observations do not communicate the hard information that is required to manage patient care. Use specific, concise terms and phrases that tell the facts and not opinion. Think about what you've observed, what you want to say, and then how you're going to say it before writing anything. This will become habit with time, but to develop the habit requires thought and effort at the start.

It is permissible to use approved abbreviations when charting, but the abbreviations must be those in general use in your program. Learn them and use them. Don't use a shorthand that nobody else can understand.

Reading

Although reading is not considered to be a direct communications skill, it is a talent that puts you in direct touch with the information and ideas you need to perform your job well. Your education from now on will depend heavily on how well and what you read. Reading is not a substitute for experience, but it is an inseparable part of your education and work. Good reading habits developed now will help you through your program and throughout your career.

How fast you read and how well you understand what you read are the essentials of effective reading. Both can be improved with practice.

How fast you read depends on what kind of material you're reading and how efficiently your eyes travel over the page. A textbook or nursing manual goes slower than a mystery story or a general-interest magazine article because of their purpose. Technical reading requires more concentration than recreational reading, but that does not mean it has to be hard. Your reading speed is also affected by how many words you read in a single glance, by whether you read each word, and by distractions such as lip reading or reading aloud.

Observe how you read. Do you mouth or speak the words? Do you keep your place by running your finger along sentences as you read? Do you read each word separately? Do you go back over what you've read again and again? Your reading speed and comprehension will suffer if you do. If you have reading problems, ask for help now. Changing poor reading habits will make learning easier.

How well you understand what you have read depends a great deal on the extent of your vocabulary. If you know the words, you will generally understand what is said, although not knowing a key word may make the rest of a sentence meaningless. An excellent way to improve comprehension is to build a good vocabulary. Nurses require two vocabularies, each with their own dictionaries: one for common language and the other for medical terms.

When you find an unfamiliar word, look it up immediately, read the definition and the correct pronunciation, repeat the word, and then say it in your own words. Then go back and read the sentence where it was found. To increase word retention and make new words a part of your active vocabulary, use them soon and frequently.

You will use medical and health terms extensively in much of your reading and in communications with colleagues and patients. Medical terminology has its own special rules, particularly regarding root words, suffixes, and prefixes. Learn them well now so that you can figure out meanings of new words on your own. Then look them up to verify your definition.

Communicating Empathy and Sympathy

As a nurse, being there for your patients will be one of your major contributions to their health. You will be in the position to give them emotional support, encouragement, and understanding. The source of this support comes from inside yourself, where your feelings reside.

Feelings require energy, and energy is a resource you cannot afford to waste. At times, just meeting the daily physical demands of your work will take more energy than you think you have. Add to that the emotional drain of working with patients who depend on you for many of their needs, and you will quickly see how the conservation of physical and emotional energy is the only way to avoid exhaustion and loss of interest.

The way to provide emotional support to your patients and not deplete your emotional reserves is to avoid becoming personally involved while still sharing with them their thoughts, feelings, and fears. It is called *empathy.*

Empathizing with someone is to project yourself into their situation to understand what they are experiencing, without experiencing it yourself. It lets you say to yourself, "How *would* I feel if I were my patient with his illness?" and not "How *do* I feel as my patient with his illness?" The latter is sympathy, which is to have another person's feelings or emotions.

Empathizing with patients lets them have their experience without interference but with the benefit of having someone who understands how important or serious it is.

Sympathizing with a patient takes away from their experience and forces them to share it with you. It is unfair to them because they, not you, must actually deal with the experience and its consequences.

Being emphathetic is not callous or hard-hearted. It lets you keep the distance you need from the patient's problem so that you can think and act in the patient's best interest.

Problem Solving

A problem is not knowing exactly what to do in a specific situation. Problems can be complex, with many parts and many consequences, or simple, with just one answer. As a nurse you will have your share of each kind of problem. Knowing how to solve them will make your job easier.

It is not a good idea to respond to a problem without thinking about it first. Although it may sometimes be faster to act without thinking, you will do better if you use a system to solve all problems to avoid making errors.

The first step to problem solving is to make sure you understand the problem. State the problem in your own words as accurately as you can. Once you know what the problem is, determine its cause. There may be more than one reason for the problem. Find as many reasons as you can before attempting a solution. Make sure your information is accurate to avoid acting on hearsay, rumor, or someone else's misinterpretation of facts.

After pinpointing the causes, see whether there is more than one solution to the problem. If so, study each to find which one will solve the problem with the least negative effect on those involved, with particular attention to your patient. Avoid letting your own motives or emotions influence the solution unless the problem is a personal one.

Once you have a solution that best fits the problem, check your institution's practices and rules to avoid conflict. Then decide who is best suited to put the solution into action.

Be careful not to use automatic solutions that are based on presumption. You may not have all the facts, or you may be seeing the problem or its solution from an inaccurate point of view. You can use your own past experiences to evaluate new problems, but avoid the trap of assuming that the solution that worked in the past will work every time. It may, but if you don't look closely at the problem, you could miss a key difference.

When you must question someone's authority to solve a problem, do so carefully. Give a clear, intelligent statement of the problem and its solution in a way that will keep the issue neutral. Problems can be worsened if the people involved are forced to defend their position or attack yours.

The following is a general guide to problem solving. Use it, but treat every problem as unique and solve each on its own merits.

Problem-Solving Hints

1. Define the problem in your own terms.
2. State your own objectives realistically.
3. Get as many facts as possible.
4. Get advice from your instructor and others if necessary.
5. Examine alternative solutions carefully.
6. Give yourself room to change solutions if necessary.
7. Choose the best solution in your judgment.
8. Take responsible action.
9. Evaluate the consequences of your action.
10. Choose another solution if your action did not solve the problem.

Discussion Questions/Learning Activities

1. List between 10 and 15 human needs and then place them in one of the five categories of human needs described by Maslow.
2. What are "first impressions" and how are they formed?
3. Describe "hidden messages" that people give by posture, appearance, and body language.
4. Think about how you might handle a situation when you know for certain that a classmate is using illegal drugs or is dependent on drugs or alcohol.
5. Describe the personal traits or characteristics that contribute to becoming an effective nurse.
6. What can you do to identify and adjust to your personal prejudices?
7. What are some effective methods you might be able to use to reduce stress and anxiety?
8. Using forms other than verbal communication, try getting a message across to a friend or classmate.
9. Select a problem related to either school or your personal life and use the problem-solving techniques presented in this chapter to find a solution(s). Did this process clarify your thinking?

Suggested Readings

Barry PD, Morgan AJ: Mental Health and Mental Illness. Philadelphia, JB Lippincott, 1985.

Gerrard B, Boniface W, Love B: Interpersonal Skills for Health Professionals. East Norwalk, CT, Appleton & Lange, 1980.

Hames CC, Joseph DH: Basic Concepts of Helping. East Norwalk, CT, Appleton & Lange, 1986.

Hood GH, Dincher JR: Total Patient Care: Foundations and Practice. St. Louis, CV Mosby, 1988.

Keane, CB: Essentials of Medical-Surgical Nursing. Philadelphia, WB Saunders, 1986.

Milliken ME: Understanding Human Behavior. Albany, NY, Delmar, 1981.

Muldarv, TW: Interpersonal Relations for Health Professionals. New York, Macmillan, 1983.

Sampson EE, Marthas M: Group Process for the Health Professions. New York, Wiley, 1981.

Shives LR, Basic Concepts of Psychiatric–Mental Health Nursing. Philadelphia, JB Lippincott, 1986.

3 Nursing From Past to Present

Objectives

When you complete this chapter, you should be able to:

Give the dates of the major historical periods and identify a significant event in each period.

Describe the contributions of Florence Nightingale to the development of modern nursing.

Trace the development of practical nursing from the late 1800s to the present time.

Name the two organizations that are primarily concerned with practical/vocational nursing education and practical/vocational nursing practice.

October 1854

The British Light Brigade was under attack at Balaklava, Turkey, by Russian troops. It was a bloody war, this war in the Crimea. Cannons blazed under the heavy gray skies of late autumn. Muskets cracked, spitting fire and sudden death. Many soldiers would die in the Crimean War. Some would die needlessly.

The British field hospital in Scutari smelled of dirt, blood, and death. Thousands of sick and wounded soldiers, many still in their blood-caked uniforms, lay helpless and cold on filthy straw beds.

The hospital was understaffed and short of supplies. Hunger and disease added to the solders' suffering. The death rate soared.

In London, 2000 miles and many days' travel away from the battle, the *London Times* told the awful story of misery at the war front. The public was outraged but felt helpless. No organized care for British victims of war yet existed.

A brave young woman offered her services. She was a nurse.

Although she had been raised in comfortable surroundings, the woman gave no thought to her own well-being or safety in volunteering to go to Turkey to care for the sick and dying. Her offer was accepted immediately.

A group of 38 women accompanied the nurse to Scutari. They were appalled by what they found. Suffering was everywhere. Wounds festered for lack of soap and clean dressings. Rats, mice, bedbugs, and lice crawled amid the moaning men, adding to their torment. To many, death was a relief—and death came to many. More than half the men were dying.

Every night the nurse walked the cold corridors to comfort the sick men. They could hear her footsteps, softly at first and then growing louder. But only when the flickering glow of her lamp brightened the darkness, did they know that the kind lady with the lamp was not a dream.

The next months were a miracle. Using her own money, the nurse bought supplies and food. The small group of dedicated women scoured the dingy hospital. The kitchen prepared hot, nutritious meals for the patients. There were organized activities for the men. The death rate decreased with astonishing speed. Six months after the women's arrival, only two percent of the patients were dying.

The courageous young nurse who volunteered her services in the Crimean War was Florence Nightingale. Her lamp, still burning brightly after 130 years, is the beacon of modern nursing.

Nursing is deeply rooted in history, even though it is relatively new as a career. Today nursing is a modern, rapidly growing, highly skilled service that is as technically sophisticated as the latest discoveries in science and medicine. But people have practiced nursing for ages, and the tradition of serving persons in need can be traced far into the past.

The historical record of nursing in very early times is vague, but the conditions for nursing have always existed. New babies, illness, injury, aging, and the need for personal care are facts of life. One can assume that people have always needed what today is called nursing.

There is also no clear record of who in a group, tribe, or society performed the functions of nursing. Modern medicine can trace its primitive origins to the skills and wisdom of witch doctors, shamans, and medicine men. They performed healing rituals and administered herbs and roots that were known for their medicinal value. Their knowledge of the natural world came from tens of thousands of years of observation and experience passed down from generation to generation. That knowledge evolved into the traditions and tools of health care as it is practiced today. Your role in nursing has been defined by long experience.

Nursing in Ancient Civilizations

As cultures developed and the civilizations based on them flourished, guidelines for behavior were made into rules. The rules were intended to protect people and guarantee group survival. They governed sanitation, hygiene, diet, sexual relations, fitness and disease, and other areas of life.

Like many early civilizations, Ancient Egypt developed on the banks of a river. Waterways such as the Nile were a source of life. But when large numbers of people lived together and used the river for drinking, washing, and sanitation, the need for personal hygiene and public sanitation became evident. Rules—early versions of community health laws—were made.

Egyptian physicians were skilled in treating fractures, filling teeth, and classifying drugs. Midwives practiced obstetrics, and friends or attendants served as nurses at births.

In ancient Babylonia, illness was seen as punishment for displeasing the gods. It was believed that atonement was possible through purifying the body with herbs and chants. Purification was performed in special temples that, in a sense, were care centers.

The Old Testament refers to many dietary, hygienic, and health laws. For example, it was forbidden to eat meat after the third day because in a hot climate without refrigeration, the meat would spoil. People with communicable diseases were isolated in sick houses. The aged were provided for. Variations of those laws are still practiced today. Health, healing, and a tradition of caring for the sick and homeless are parts of an ancient heritage that continues.

Other very early cultures practiced health and healing principles that were also forerunners of today's medicine and nursing. Over 3000 years ago, the *Vedas* (sacred Hindu books of India's earliest cultures) told of major and minor surgery, nervous afflictions, and urinary system diseases. Later in India, advances were made in medicine, surgery, prenatal care, hygiene, and sanitation. They included public hospitals that were staffed by male nurses who would be qualified by today's standards to be practical nurses.

In ancient China, acupuncture, medical diagnosis by a complex pulse theory, and a vast knowledge of medicine and drugs were well known. This knowledge has survived and in various forms is still practiced today.

A physician of the late fifth century B.C. named Hippocrates (460–370 B.C.) is referred to by early Greek writers as the "Father of Medicine." He is still called that today. He taught at a medical school on Cos, a small Greek island. Little is known of his ideas and discoveries, and much of his life is unknown. The Hippocratic oath, which is taken by medical school graduates today, is attributed to Hippocrates.

The rise of the teachings of the school at Cos and another at Cnidus ended the dominance that magic held in early medicine. The study of medicine shifted to a more scientific course.

Hippocrates' followers said diseases always had specific causes. They believed that the causes could be discovered by examination and analysis. The causes they sought were often wrong—they blamed disease on "humors" in the body, such as blood, phlegm, and yellow and black bile.

The idea that it is not magic or wrongdoing that causes illness was a big step forward. *Diagnosis* (the process of identifying a disease or medical condition scientifically) and *prognosis* (predicting the probable outcome of a patient's disease), rather than *cure* (the restoration to health), were the foundations of Hippocratic medicine. It would be more than 2000 years later that scientists would discover the germ theory of disease (much disease is caused by microorganisms).

The healing method taught by Hippocrates' followers was to help nature do its work. This was similar to what Florence Nightingale would write about nursing in her *Notes on Nursing: What It Is and What It Is Not* in 1859, more than 2000 years later. She said that nursing would "put the patient in the best condition for nature to act upon."

Practitioners of Hippocratic medicine were men who did not train nurses to do the nursing that their method—"help nature do its work"—suggested. They did it themselves. Women in Greek society were subordinate to men. It was believed that women were not worthy of medical or nursing education. Greek nurses were little more than household servants—usually slaves—who took care of the children and family.

The rise of the vast Roman Empire (27 B.C. to A.D. 476) was based on military might. Military hospitals to care for wounded soldiers were established, but Roman medicine was still based on superstition. This was a setback from advances made earlier by the Greeks. The Romans held their women in greater esteem than the Greeks did theirs. Roman women enjoyed a liberated position for the times, but organized nursing care was not yet established.

Nursing in the Early Christian Era (First to Fifth Centuries A.D.)

Nursing by women who were dedicated to its practice began with the acceptance of Christianity, which taught caring for others. Deacons and deaconesses—men and women with equal rank in the church—served the sick, the poor, the aged, orphans, widows, slaves, and prisoners. They fed and clothed the needy, cared for the sick, visited prisoners, sheltered the homeless, and buried the dead. All were works of mercy.

Deaconesses were frequently well-bred, cultured widows or daughters of Roman officials. They performed services similar to today's community health or visiting nurses, carrying baskets of food and medicine to needy homes. Phoebe, who lived about A.D. 55, is considered to be the first deaconess and visiting nurse. She is mentioned in the New Testament.

Two other women's groups, the Order of Widows and the Order of Virgins, were also dedicated to the principle of merciful care for those in need. Like the deaconesses, they lived in humble, selfless service to others. They are sometimes called the first organized public health service nurses.

The deaconess movement reached its peak at about A.D. 400 in Constantinople (today's Istanbul, Turkey), which was an important center of the early Christian church. The movement diminished when the church took away the role of the deaconesses, but not before spreading as far west as present-day France and Ireland.

In A.D. 380 in Rome, a beautiful and wealthy woman named Fabiola founded the first public hospital. She had divorced her first husband and was remarried when she converted to Christianity. Her second husband died. Because remarriage after divorce was considered a sin, Fabiola atoned by dedicating her life to charity. To the dismay of others, she personally cared for the sick and injured, often cleaning and dressing sores and wounds with her own hands.

The Dark Ages and the Monastic Orders (A.D. 476 to 1000)

The influence of the Roman Empire peaked at the time of the birth of Jesus. It ended in A.D. 476, after hundreds of years of attacks by barbarians. Europe was split into many separate kingdoms. The next 500 years are called the Dark Ages because learning almost stopped. Christians retreated to walled monasteries while the world was plunged into war, rivalry, and ignorance. The teachings of the early Greek Classical period were saved by the dedication of monks who lived in relative safety in monasteries. They kept learning alive and preserved the record of the past in handwritten books.

The idea of caring for those in need was also preserved. The emphasis in medicine shifted from a scientific interest in anatomy, physiology, and the healing effects of nature's drugs to personal care and comfort, which is the foundation of nursing. Monks and nuns performed nursing tasks in the monasteries under the direction of the church.

The first hospitals were founded at monasteries in Lyon in A.D. 542 and Paris in A.D. 650. Santo Spiritu Hospital was founded in Rome in A.D. 717. The first nursing order of nuns, the Augustinian Sisters, staffed the hospital in Paris.

The Middle Ages (1000-1450)

The small states that emerged from the Dark Ages were dominated by the church, which had slowly filled the vacuum left by the collapse of the Roman Empire. Almost everything in life, from philosophy, politics, art, and architecture to everyday activity, was deeply influenced by the church.

During this time, huge cathedrals were built and universities were founded. Some of the universities are still in existence today. A lengthy series of religious wars, the Crusades, began.

The Dark Ages had closed off much of Western civilization for almost 500 years. The Crusades reopened it.

The Crusaders were military orders of priests, brothers, and knights who sought to reclaim the Holy Land from the Moslems.

The Moslems used organized facilities for the care of their sick and wounded. The Crusaders saw this and adopted this method of treatment to care for their own casualties. They built hospitals near the battlefields. While some knights fought on the battlefield, others cared for the injured in the hospitals. The insignia of the Knights Hospitalers of St. John of Jerusalem, also known as Knights Hospitalers, was a bright red cross. It is now the symbol of the International Red Cross.

The Knights Hospitalers' strict principles of discipline, obedience, and devotion became an important part of organized nursing for hundreds of years. Knights who returned home from the wars in the Holy Land created a new version of society based on a middle class. The deaconess movement vanished and was replaced by monastic nursing orders such as the Franciscans, the Alexians, the Brothers of Mercy, and the Knights of St. John, a military order that was formed to fight the Crusades.

Monasteries continued to play an important role in nursing during the Middle Ages. Hospices were established within their walls. As places of safety from the outside world, the hospices welcomed travelers, the poor, and the sick. The idea of separate hospitals for the sick was begun later. They were based on the hospitals of the Persians and Arabs, whose ideas were brought back to Europe by the Crusaders. The hospitals were staffed by both secular and religious orders.

Two early orders are still active. The First Order of St. Francis and the Second Order of St. Francis were regular monastic orders. Order members lived secluded lives under strict vows of poverty and chastity. The First Order of St. Francis was founded by Saint Francis of Assisi. The Second Order, now called the Poor Clares, was founded by his disciple, St. Clare. St. Francis also founded the Third Order of St. Francis for laypersons who wanted to follow his teachings but did not want to give up normal life for the strict discipline of the monastery. The Poor Clares continue to serve the poor and the aged today, but they do not perform nursing functions.

Nursing during the Middle Ages was an important way of life to its practitioners and a valuable service to those in need. Its practice reinforced its place in the slowly growing science of medicine. Its strict organization was also important. When new members joined nursing orders, they first had to spend a probationary period before they could wear the white robe that symbolized their work. After an additional novitiate period, they were allowed to wear the hood of the order. A nursing director, called a *maitresse,* supervised their activities. Order members were expected to be obedient, unselfish, and totally devoted to the performance of their duties. These and other regulations are the roots of traditional nursing.

During this time the power of the Catholic Church grew. Because the church was the sponsor of the nursing orders, the orders' strength and status also grew. The numbers of women entering nursing increased. Nursing was a popular and acceptable occupation for women.

At the same time, medicine as an occupation declined. The church did not favor medicine in the way it did nursing. The church, not medicine, held authority over nursing. What a nurse could and could not do was dictated by the church. For example, because it was believed that the human body was basically unclean, procedures such as perineal care, enemas, and douches were not performed. A nurse's priority was to serve her patients' spiritual needs. However, her duties included feeding, bathing, and washing patients, administering medications, changing dressing and linens, and all-around cleaning.

The nurse, not the physician, provided most health care in hospitals, even though the care was more custodial and centered on reducing discomfort than treatment centered.

The church's authority and dominance began to decline. The kingdoms that were formed after the end of the Roman empire grew in power. The crusaders had returned to Europe with ideas from the Moslem world and ancient Greece. They also brought the deadly plague, a highly contagious, epidemic disease. In the 1300s, plague swept Europe. One fourth of the entire population died. Famines and war killed many more people. Economies faltered. With such chaos affecting their lives, people's religious fervor turned to cynicism and lost hope. The times were ripe for change.

The Decline of Nursing: The Renaissance (1400–1600) to the Nineteenth Century

An Augustinian monk named Martin Luther opposed many of the teachings of the Catholic Church. His protests led to the Reformation and the foundation of a new view of religion, Protestantism ended the absolute domination of the Catholic Church. It also opened the way for new ideas in areas other than religion. Some had a dramatic effect on nursing.

Monasteries were closed. The religious orders that ran them were disbanded. Nursing work once performed by women in hospitals virtually stopped. The role of women in society changed dramatically.

Under the influence of the church, women had been revered. They were encouraged to do charitable work outside the home. Women from Europe's finest families had became nuns who taught and nursed.

Under Protestantism, women were considered to be subordinate to men. They were expected to stay at home to bear and raise children and to care for the home. Respectable women did not work in hospitals. Instead, nursing was done by "wayward" women of low status, such as prostitutes and alcoholic women who were given the work in place of going to jail.

Nursing fell to a low state, and its practitioners were reduced to poorly paid servants. The disruption of society by plague and famine meant that there were more sick and poor persons than ever.

The early Greeks and Romans had developed wonderful ideas, but the ideas had been lost for centuries. Now the ideas were replanted. In a burst of collective creative genius known as the Renaissance—meaning *rebirth*—that lasted until the sixteenth century, classical thought was raised to near perfection. The idea that the world could be studied became the foundation of a new science of discovery and exploration. That idea is still alive today.

Medicine took a lead among the sciences. Anatomy, physiology, and the scientific basis of healing were studied. Nursing went into a further decline.

Nursing had been neglected during the Greek era, when Hippocratic medicine prevailed. It rose to dominate medicine during the monastic period. Now, during the Renaissance, it fell once again. Except for the hope represented by dedicated people such as St. Vincent de Paul, a French priest who, with follower Louise de Marilac, founded the Sisters of Charity, nursing remained dormant until the early 1820s.

The Emergence of Modern Nursing (Nineteenth Century)

Social conditions had deteriorated sharply by the end of the 1700s. Industrialization was replacing familiar agricultural society. Cities with large populations were breeding grounds for poverty, poor hygiene, and disease. Societies treated their members badly. The sick, insane, poor, and homeless were put into hospitals, jails, asylums, and poorhouses that were little more than warehouses for the needy. Living, health, and sanitary conditions were deplorable. Change was desperately needed. The stage for social reform was set. All that was needed were people with social vision.

A Londoner, John Howard (1726-1790), fought for reforms in public health. He had visited many foreign countries. He had seen at first hand how prisoners were treated. He pushed for prison reforms that resulted in dramatic improvements in prison conditions and increased public awareness.

Howard's work was carried on by a London philanthropist, Elizabeth Fry (1780–1845). She organized a group called the Protestant Sisters of Charity, later called the Institute of Nursing Sisters, to provide nursing care for London's poor.

In Germany, a minister in Kaiserswerth was concerned with the problems of poverty faced by his parishoners. Pastor Theodor Fliedner (1800–1864) visited England, where he was impressed by Elizabeth Fry's work in British prisons. With his wife, Friederike, Fliedner opened a school in Germany to train deaconesses, the Kaiserswerth Deaconess Institution. It marked a revival of the deaconess movement that had ended 400 years earlier. It was the first real nursing school.

Pastor Fliedner opened his hospital in Kaiserswerth in 1836. Its first deaconess was Gertrude Reichardt. Many women were trained as deaconesses at the school. They became the core of the movement that would lead to modern nursing. Graduates of the Kaiserswerth Deaconess Institution founded similar programs to train women around the world.

One of them, Florence Nightingale, opened the way to the new age of nursing.

Florence Nightingale (1820–1910)

Florence Nightingale was the younger of two sisters. She was born on May 13, 1820, in Florence, Italy, and was named after that city. Her parents were visiting there from their native England. She returned to England with her family when she was a year old. As a daughter of wealthy parents, she was given an excellent classical education in languages, history, mathematics, and philosophy. She was taught the social manners and customs of the privileged class and grew up to be a cultured, attractive young lady. Her family expected her to become the wife of an equally eminent gentleman and live a life of comfort and plenty. Her own goals were decidedly different.

From childhood on, Miss Nightingale was a sympathetic and sensitive girl with a great affection for animals and people. As a youngster she visited the sick and poor. Her visits were a hint of her growing ambition to serve humanity. She began to think of a career as a nurse. She declared her intentions in 1844, when she was 24 years old.

The idea astounded her parents. Not only did such work not fit her social rank, but at that time women in nursing were often disreputable. The more her family objected to her calling, as she believed it to be, the more determined she became.

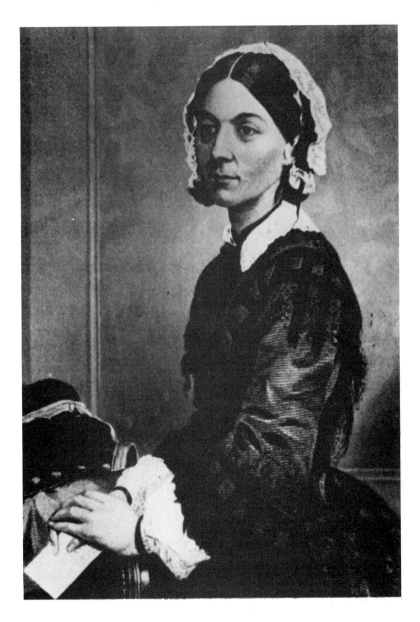

Modern nursing began with Florence Nightingale. (Courtesy of The Center for the Study of the History of Nursing.)

Miss Nightingale traveled to foreign countries. She visited hospitals and orphanages where she observed how nursing was performed by untrained individuals. She became an authority on public health and hospitals.

Dr. Elizabeth Blackwell, a close friend who was also America's first woman physician, encouraged Miss Nightingale to pursue her ambition to be a nurse.

In 1851, at 31 years of age, Florence Nightingale went to the Kaisers-werth Deaconess Institution, which she had heard about from friends. She studied there for 3 months. After her training, she worked in Paris with the Sisters of Charity. She also observed skilled French surgeons operate. Although she was pleased with her training, she knew it was not enough for the kind of nurse she wanted to be.

Florence returned to London, where she became superintendent of a small institution, the Establishment for Gentlewomen During Illness. Her family had still not accepted her independent attitude. Then, in 1854, the Crimean War broke out. This dark moment of history would certify her behavior. It would also help her leave her mark on the world from then on.

British newspapers told of appalling conditions in the Crimea, where England, France, and Turkey were fighting against Russia. Ill and injured British soldiers lay neglected, while both allied and enemy soldiers were treated and cared for by organized groups of nurses. French casualties were taken care of by the Sisters of Charity. The Russians were cared for by the Sisters of Mercy. The English public was outraged. Miss Nightingale volunteered to take a group of nurses to the Crimea to care for English and Turkish soldiers. Her friend Sidney Herbert, Britain's secretary of war, had already written to her requesting her services.

On October 21, 1854, Florence Nightingale went to the front with 38 women. Some were trained as nurses, and others were not. They took with them a stock of badly needed supplies.

Conditions at the front were disgusting. Wounded soldiers, still in bloody uniforms, lay crowded into filthy wards on dirty straw. Sanitation was poor to nonexistent. There was no soap, clean linen, or even tables and chairs. The food was often inedible. Adding to the horror, the reception the women received from army medical officers was characterized by resentment.

Miss Nightingale took matters into her own hands. With her nurses, she tended to ill and injured soldiers. She fought red tape to obtain supplies. She hired people to clean the hospitals. She set up laundries. She organized kitchens to turn out nutritious meals. She personally made endless rounds to comfort wounded and sick soldiers. She even used her own money to purchase supplies.

Within 6 months, Florence Nightingale's labors paid off. Deaths dropped dramatically, from 420 per 1000 to 22 per 1000. Discipline and organization took over from neglect and disorder. She had become the

"Lady with the Lamp" to her patients. It was an endearing reference to the nightly rounds she made with a lamp in hand to see to their comfort and care.

Florence Nightingale returned to England in July 1856. She was the unchallenged heroine of the war. But her own strength was sapped by sickness and exhaustion. She remained a semiinvalid for the remaining 54 years of her life.

Florence Nightingale did not stop her work, however. Her powerful influence was felt in civilian and military hospitals and in nurse training. She also wrote books. Her best-known work is *Notes on Nursing: What It Is and What It Is Not.* She was awarded medals and jewels by grateful admirers who included England's Queen Victoria and the sultan of Turkey. A fund contributed by soldiers and citizens alike was used to establish a training school for nurses, the Nightingale School, which opened in 1860. The school became the model for modern nursing schools. Florence Nightingale died in 1910 at 90 years of age.

Nursing During the Late Nineteenth and Early Twentieth Centuries (1890–1960)

Nursing was changed forever by Florence Nightingale and the methods she introduced. Much of the world remained in the "dark ages" of nursing care, and the need for nursing remained the same since time began. At last, with a proven method to tend to that need, modern nursing could supply new practices of care that would carry nursing into the future. The old practices fell away as major advances in nursing were made around the world.

The International Red Cross was founded in Switzerland in 1864 by J. H. Dunant. Like Florence Nightingale, Dunant had been horrified by the almost complete lack of care for the sick and wounded in wartime. Until that time there was no neutral international health organization that nations could turn to in time of war or after natural disasters. One of the Red Cross's early accomplishments was to make rules for the treatment of the wounded and for the protection of medical personnel and hospitals. They are called the Geneva Convention.

The American Red Cross was formed in 1881 by Clara Barton to serve the United States. It was similar to the international body. Other countries formed their own organizations.

There were no formal programs to train nurses, and there were scarcely any trained nurses at all in the United States. War and other social conditions were major influences in the reform of the haphazard nursing practices that did exist. Government agencies became aware of the problem, and important changes were made. The Civil War (1861–1865) dramatized the need for skilled nurses. People realized that society was responsible for its own health. The status of women was improving, and Florence Nightingale's example led to advances in nursing education and practice.

Women were beginning to assume new roles in public affairs, including nursing. In New York City, Bellevue Hospital opened the New York Training School in 1873, which was organized along the lines of the Nightingale School model.

Fifteen years later the Mills School of Nursing, a school for training male nurses, was opened at Bellevue Hospital. Other schools were opened as the new nursing movement grew. Textbooks, uniforms for secular nurses, and a growing appreciation of nurses by a grateful public for their devotion to duty encouraged the growth.

Science and medicine made gigantic strides. The germ theory of disease was developed in 1876 by Robert Koch, a German bacteriologist. He said that bacteria, not "bad air," carry anthrax and other diseases. Louis Pasteur's discoveries in chemistry and microbiology (pasteurization is named for him), Joseph Lister's aseptic surgical techniques, Ignaz Philipp Semmelweis's conquest of puerpural sepsis (childbed fever), and other scientific developments were changing humankind's inability to do something about its health.

Nursing also flourished. A number of eminent women emerged as leaders of the growing reform.

Dorothea Lynde Dix (1802–1887) was concerned by the inhumane treatment of mentally ill persons. She traveled over the United States to encourage legislators to pass protective laws. As an untrained volunteer nurse in the Civil War, she was appointed to be superintendent of women nurses for all military hospitals. She was the first U.S. Army nurse.

Clara Barton (1821–1912) was a dedicated teacher at a time when very few women held such jobs. She obtained permission from the U.S. government to take volunteer nursing to field hospitals during the Civil War. She cared for the ill and wounded of both sides, North and South, black and white, with equality. She was given the name "Angel of the Battlefield." Miss Barton formed the American Association of the Red Cross in 1881 after reading about the awful conditions of soldiers on the battlefield.

The first nurse to be trained in the United States was Linda Richards (1841–1930), who graduated from the New England Hospital for Women and Children, in Boston, after a 1-year training program. She developed a system for writing accurate patient reports that later became the basis for nursing and hospital record keeping. She was a lifelong student of nursing and taught its methods. She traveled extensively, studying, lecturing, consulting, and opening schools. The Linda Richards Award is given every 2 years by the National League for Nursing (NLN) to an active nurse who has significantly contributed to nursing.

There are others who stand out in American nursing history.

Isabel Hampton Robb (1860–1910) advocated nurses' rights, a 3-year training program, 8-hour instead of 12-hour workdays, and licensure to protect patients.

Lavinia Dock (1858–1956) was instrumental in the beginning of what is now called the National League for Nursing. Her book, *History of Nursing*, coauthored with Mary Adelaide Nutting, is the classic text on the subject.

Mary Eliza Mahoney (1845–1926) was the first black graduate professional nurse in the United States. Her work for integration in nursing and improved working and health care conditions was a lifelong endeavor. The Mary Mahoney Award, first instituted in 1936, is given by the American Nurses' Association to recognize her accomplishments.

Lillian Wald (1867–1940) opened public health nursing in the United States when she founded the Henry Street Settlement in 1893 to provide free nursing care for the poor on the Lower East Side of New York City.

Mary Adelaide Nutting (1858–1947) graduated from the first class of the Johns Hopkins School of Nursing. She founded the first college-level department of nursing at Columbia University Teacher's College and was instrumental in raising the standards of nursing education. She wrote the four-volume *History of Nursing* with Lavinia Dock.

Annie W. Goodrich (1876–1955) was a strong-willed advocate of nursing training and the need to raise nursing to professional status. When World War I created the need for more nurses, she wrote plans for the Army School of Nursing.

Clara Maass (1876–1901) was a former volunteer contract nurse with the U.S. Army. She gave her life in an experiment to discover the cause of yellow fever. As a test subject, she was infected twice by mosquito bites and died at 25 years of age.

As the need for nurses, appropriate training, and better standards grew through the years, the American nursing community produced dedicated members to meet each demand. The number of nurses has risen during times of national emergency and war. In less critical times the number has fallen. But there is always a need for well-trained, qualified nurses in good times and bad.

To provide care for patients at any time, the health care team needs competent, intelligent practitioners. An important member of this team is the practical/vocational nurse.

The Development of Practical/Vocational Nursing

Before the 1860s and the foundation of professional nursing schools, nursing in America was done by practical nurses who learned by experience rather than by formal education. The nursing schools that opened in the last half of the nineteenth century changed that. Professional nurses have been educated in formal programs ever since. Practical nursing education has had a similar history, although the formal education programs came somewhat later.

The Industrial Revolution of the mid-1800s began a population shift from rural to urban areas of the United States. It is still going on today. In the last century, many of the people who left the farm for the city were untrained. Very often they were also uneducated.

The young women who arrived in the cities were particularly disadvantaged because there were few job opportunities for them. Men could find work in factories, but women were limited to domestic service.

To train women so that they could increase their opportunity to compete for jobs, the Young Women's Christian Association (YWCA), a church-affiliated organization that originated in Europe, gave classes in cooking and domestic chores. It is likely that simple home nursing skills and child care instruction were included.

In 1892 a formal 3-month YWCA course in practical nursing was offered for the first time in the United States, in Brooklyn, New York. Its objective was to teach practical nurses how to care for children, invalids, and the elderly. Practical nurses were often in demand to fill nursing shortages. The Ballard School, named for its sponsor, Miss Lucinda Ballard, was a response to the need for a system to educate them.

Fifteen years later, in 1907, the Thompson School in Brattleboro, Vermont, was opened. In 1918 the Household Nursing Association School of Attendant Nursing was founded in Boston. The objective of the programs at these schools was to train practical nurses in home nursing skills. The training emphasized cooking, cleaning, and other household duties. Some early practical nursing programs also provided hospital experience. If the program was affiliated with a hospital, it paid its students for their services. These programs were the models for today's schools of practical nursing. Household Nursing was renamed the Shephard-Gill School of Practical Nursing. The Ballard School closed in 1948 after more than a half century of success. Shepherd-Gill School and the Thompson School are still in operation.

There were few controls, little educational planning, and minimum supervision of practical nursing schools before 1940. Standards were non-existent and the programs varied widely. It was only after state agencies that were subject to legislation took over that controls were established. Although Mississippi required mandatory licensing for practical nurses in 1914, and the Minneapolis Girls' Vocational High School offered the first vocational school practical nurse program in 1919, it was not until 1941 that a national association for practical nursing was formed.

The Association of Practical Nurse Schools was organized in Chicago in 1941 to address the needs of practical nursing education. Hilda M. Torrop, the director of the Ballard School, Etta Creech, the director of the Family Health Association, in Cleveland, and Katherine Shephard, the executive director of the Household Nursing Association, in Boston, were the association's officers. Its name was changed to the National Association of Practical Nurse Education (NAPNE) in 1942, when membership was opened to practical nurses.

A service for accrediting practical nursing schools was begun by the association in 1945. This service was ended in 1984. In 1959 it organized a summer school and workshops for directors and instructors of practical nursing programs. Its journal, the first one for practical nursing and now called *The Journal of Practical Nursing,* was begun in 1951.

The association changed its name in 1959 to the National Association for Practical Nurse Education and Service (NAPNES). By then it was sponsoring summer courses at colleges and universities, was emphasizing continuing education for practical nurses and their welfare, and had established a Department of Education and a Department of Service to State Practical Nursing Associations. Membership in the NAPNES is open to anyone who is interested in promoting the interests, concerns, and occupation of practical nursing.

In 1949, Lillian Kuster organized, and became the executive director of, the National Federation of Licensed Practical Nurses (NFLPN), the official membership organization for licensed practical and vocational nurses. Membership in NFLPN is limited to licensed practical and vocational nurses.

These two organizations, NAPNES and NFLPN, educate and inform the general public about practical nursing, its programs, and licensure requirements.

Discussion Questions/Learning Activities

1. Discuss how the changing role and status of women may have influenced the development of nursing.
2. Identify some of the personal characteristics of the nurses who made important contributions to nursing between 1890 and 1900.
3. Use library resources to explore in detail the contributions of a particular nurse.
4. Write to NAPNES and NFLPN to obtain information on membership in these organizations.
5. Compare early practical nursing journal articles with articles in current journals. Try to identify changes in the articles in these journals that reflect changes in practical nursing.

References

Dolan JA: Nursing in Society: A Historical Perspective. Philadelphia, WB Saunders, 1983.

Donahue MP: Nursing: The Finest Art. St. Louis, CV Mosby, 1985.

Ellis JR, Hartley CL: Nursing in Today's World: Challenges, Issues, and Trends. Philadelphia, JB Lippincott, 1988.

Fitzpatrick ML: Prologue to Professionalism. East Norwalk, CT, Appleton & Lange, 1983.

James J, Reverby S (eds.): A Livinia Dock Reader. New York: Garland, 1985.

Kalisch BJ, Kalisch PA: The Advance of American Nursing. Boston, Little, Brown, 1986.

Nightingale F: Notes on Nursing. Philadelphia, JB Lippincott, 1859 (reproduction).

Stewart IM, Austin AL: A History of Nursing. New York, GP Putnam's Sons, 1962.

Practical/Vocational Nursing Education

4

Objectives

When you complete this chapter, you should be able to:

Explain the difference between "professional" and "nonprofessional" in terms of education.

Describe the educational preparation for registered nurses.

Describe the educational preparation for practical/vocational nurses.

List at least three types of institutions that can sponsor practical/vocational nursing programs.

Explain the difference between the terms "program approval" and "program accreditation."

Paraphrase the major points of either the NFLPN or NAPNES Standards for practical/vocational nurses.

Describe the procedure for obtaining a license as a practical/vocational nurse.

List some of the reasons why a nursing license can be suspended or revoked.

It was Rose's first visit to her high school since her graduation a few years earlier. She breathed deeply as she opened the door of the red brick building. The familiar smells of oiled wood floors and pine cleaner assaulted her nostrils. The long rows of lockers still lined the hallway. Even the paint on the walls was the same color. Nothing had changed.

Suddenly the hall was filled with girls and boys rushing to their classes. She watched them hurry by. Then the metallic clang of a bell sounded and, as if by magic, the long hall became deserted.

Rose walked slowly down the hall. She knew exactly where she was going. "Locker 213," she said aloud. There was her old locker, nestled against the wall in a line of others that had seemed a mile long when she used to run to it between bells.

"*Rose?*"

A woman in a nurse's uniform threw her arms around Rose. "Terri!" laughed Rose. She hugged the woman tightly. They had been classmates in this very school.

"Come to my office," Terri said, "so we can talk."

Rose looked around the tidy office. A student lay on a cot with a thermometer in her mouth. A boy was weighing himself on a scale in the corner. A nurse was talking to the boy. Rose turned to Terri. "Remember how I wanted to be a nurse when we were in school?" she said. "Now it's too late. I've got two kids . . ."

Terri smiled. "So do I," she said. "and I've been a nurse for only 2 years. I went back to school 3 years ago and . . ."

Rose rubbed her eyes. "It only takes 1 year to be a nurse?" she asked.

"One year of *hard work,*" Terri said. "I'm a licensed practical nurse," she added proudly. "And you can be, too, if you really want to be."

"I do!" Rose said excitedly. "But how? Tell me all about it."

It would take more than a short meeting in a busy nurse's schedule to describe practical/vocational nursing today. The vocation has come a long way since the first school of practical nursing in the United States opened in 1892. The YWCA program at the Ballard School in New York was a mere 3 months long.

Other programs to educate nonprofessional nurses and nurse's assistants, such as those developed to train Red Cross nurse's aides in World Wars I and II, were also short. For example, the World War II program consisted of only 35 hours of lecture and 45 hours of supervised clinical experience.

It was already clear that there was a permanent place for practical nurses in American health care. A number of schools were in operation, but before 1940 they operated with minimal educational planning and supervision. With the establishment of a practical nurse association—the National Association of Practical Nurse Education (NAPNE), now known as the National Association for Practical Nurse Education and Service, Inc. (NAPNES)—in the 1940s to regulate education and practice, the programs for training nonprofessional nurses became more nearly uniform. Laws for certification and licensure were also established, so that today, virtually every program in every state is governed by regulating agencies.

Defining "Professional" and "Nonprofessional"

The term "professional" generally implies someone who is competent and qualified to perform a specific occupation. Examples are professional electrician, professional secretary, and professional painter. In this context the term professional refers to someone who is an expert in his occupation. When someone refers to a person as "a real professional," it means that the person approaches the occupation with seriousness, has a high level of integrity, and can be trusted to maintain high personal standards when performing that occupation.

When the term professional is used in education, it has a somewhat different meaning. A professional education requires a minimum of 4-years of college; more often, a total of 6 or 8 years of formal study beyond high school is required. A person who studies theory and the application of theory in a specific occupation, subscribes to an occupational code of ethics, participates in the development of the occupation through organizational activities and research, and works independently of others is a professional.

The term "nonprofessional," therefore, refers only to a nurse's educational preparation. All nurses should approach their responsibilities with a professional attitude. That is, any nurse, regardless of educational preparation, should be serious about the occupation, have a high level of integrity, be trustworthy, and maintain high standards.

Types of Nursing Programs

Four-year Professional Nursing Programs

A professional nurse is one who has completed at least 4 years of college and has passed the registered nurse licensure examination. He or she has studied nursing theory and its application to practice, performs responsibilities according to a strict code of ethics, and participates in the development of nursing through membership in nursing organizations. In addition, the professional nurse engages in research in nursing and often works independently—without direct supervision. Many registered nurses who have completed a professional nursing education program have advanced to positions of leadership in nursing education and nursing service.

Two-year Associate Degree Programs

The nurse who prepares for the occupation of nursing in 2 years and passes the registered nurse licensure examination is sometimes called an associate-degree or a technical nurse. These 2-year programs are sponsored by community, technical, and junior colleges. The development of 2-year nursing programs has grown rapidly since the first programs were established by Mildred Montag in 1952. In 1974 there were 1372 2-year programs, and in 1983 there were 1490 2-year programs.

Diploma Nursing Programs

Nursing education programs sponsored by hospitals are called diploma nursing programs. These programs vary in length from 2 to 3 years. Graduates of these programs who pass the registered nurse licensure examination are sometimes called diploma nurses. The programs of study vary greatly; however, the emphasis is on developing skills in clinical nursing practice.

Practical/Vocational Nursing Programs

A practical nurse is prepared for the occupation of practical nursing in approximately one year. Practical nursing programs may be sponsored by vocational or technical schools, community or junior colleges, or hospitals. The emphasis in practical/vocational nursing education is on learning basic nursing skills that can be applied to patients in a variety of health care settings. The practical/vocational nurse, in most health care situations, functions under the supervision and direction of a registered nurse. In 1983 there were 1323 schools of practical nursing with a total enrollment of 57,011 students. In that same year there were 781,506 people holding licenses as practical or vocational nurses.

Educational requirements to become a practical/vocational nurse vary from state to state; however, most adult programs are between 10 and 18 months in length. Practical/vocational nursing programs are classified as adult practical/vocational nursing programs if the program is for adults and is not part of a high school curriculum. High school practical/vocational nursing programs are those offered to high school students. Extended high school programs require additional time in school after high school graduation.

A number of sponsoring institutions administer practical nursing/vocational programs. They include trade, technical, and vocational schools, colleges and universities, junior and community colleges, hospitals, and private or government agencies. All programs are approved by their state board of nursing.

The philosophy, objectives, and curriculum of a practical/vocational nursing program are developed by the faculty. This basic framework of your educational program is periodically reviewed, evaluated, and revised by the faculty to ensure a program of instruction that will prepare you for your first position as a practical/vocational nurse.

Since most changes in philosophy, objectives, and curriculum proposed by the faculty of a practical/vocational nursing program must first be approved by the state board of nursing, it is important to understand the approval and accreditation process.

Approval and Accreditation

Each state has a board of nursing composed of nurses, consumers, and others interested in health care. It is this organization that is responsible for nursing services to citizens within its jurisdiction. As part of their responsibility for safeguarding the well-being of their constituents, the various state boards of nursing evaluate and approve nursing education programs within their state. Schools or organizations offering nursing programs must have the approval of the state board of nursing to operate nursing education programs. Part of the approval process includes specific regulations governing the length (in hours) of nursing education programs. Graduation from a state-approved school of practical/vocational nursing is one of the prerequisites for taking the practical/vocational nursing licensing examination.

In addition to mandatory approval by the state board of nursing, many schools voluntarily seek accreditation from the National League for Nursing (NLN). The key words "approval" and "accreditation" are essential to understanding the difference between the purpose of the state board of nursing and the purpose of the NLN. Approval by the state board of nursing is mandatory; accreditation by the NLN is voluntary.

Accreditation of a program by the NLN is often an indication that a particular nursing education program exceeds the minimum requirements for conducting a program. This does not imply, however, that programs not accredited by the NLN do not exceed the minimum standards established by a state board of nursing. Since the accreditation process is voluntary, some schools, for their own unique reasons, do not seek NLN accreditation. The nonaccredited program may exceed minimum standards by far, and it may offer an outstanding education program. One must be careful when using the term "approval," which is required, and the term "accreditation," which is voluntary, when discussing the quality of a nursing education program.

Your school may be scheduled for a program review by the state board of nursing or the NLN during the time you are enrolled. Having an approval or accreditation visit is a very important process and one in which your participation will be expected.

Program Curriculum and Objectives

Generally, the early practical/vocational nursing programs were combined courses of theoretical (classroom) and clinical (institution) instruction that took approximately 2000 hours or 1 year to complete. The classroom phase took about one third of that time and consisted of lecture and laboratory classes. The remainder of the course was given to the clinical phase, with supervised experience in approved hospitals and institutions, in combination with some home care nursing experience.

It is no longer believed that classroom instruction, followed by clinical instruction, is educationally sound. The trend today is to relate classroom theory, laboratory practice, and clinical experience by offering integrated

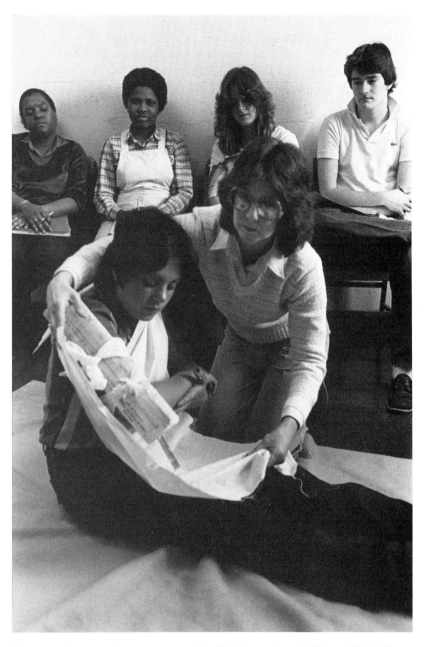

Classroom demonstrations prepare you for clinical practice. (© Richard Wood, Taurus Photos.)

sections over the length of the entire program. However, there is considerable variety in the actual organization of individual programs around the country in this regard, just as there is in the specific courses that are offered.

A typical program starts in the fall (or first semester) with an introduction to basic nursing. Subjects covered through the year include fundamentals of nursing, communication skills, anatomy and physiology, nutrition, mental health, microbiology, maternity nursing, medical and surgical nursing of adults and children, pediatrics, diet therapy, pharmacology, and geriatrics. Elective courses in the humanities and the behavioral sciences may also be offered. Teaching is by individual instructors or teams.

On successful completion of a licensed practical/vocational nursing course, a graduate should have the following:

1. The education and experience needed to qualify for and pass the licensing exam for LP/VNs in the candidate's own state.
2. The knowledge and skills to perform entry level-tasks under appropriate supervision as a licensed practical/vocational nurse.
3. The knowledge and skills to help to meet a patient's needs, including physical, emotional, social, and spiritual requirements.
4. Up-to-date information about health and disease prevention to teach to the community at large as a member of a local health care team.
5. Familiarity with social, medical, health, and technological change.
6. Awareness of local and national practical/vocational nurse associations and what they do.
7. A desire to continue the process of learning and growing in the field.

Standards for the Licensed Practical/Vocational Nurse

Two national organizations are primarily concerned with the practice of practical nursing. Membership in the National Federation of Licensed Practical Nurses (NFLPN) is only open to licensed practical/vocational nurses (LP/VNs). The National Association for Practical Nurse Education and Service (NAPNES) accepts for membership anyone who is interested in promoting the practice of practical/vocational nursing. Both national organizations have issued statements that define the standard of nursing that should be expected from a LP/VN.

In 1970 the NFLPN approved the "Statement of Functions and Qualifications of the Licensed Practical Nurse," which was written to help clarify an LPN's responsibilities. It was revised in 1972 and again in 1979. In 1987, that statement was replaced by a new statement entitled "Nursing Practice Standards for the Licensed Practical/Vocational Nurse."

The new statement defined LP/VN nursing practice standards in its preface as a model for measuring and evaluating the quality of health services and nursing care by LP/VNs in any practice setting, including specialized nursing services individually applied according to patient need, type of agency or service, and community resources. The full text of this statement is in Appendix D. This document basically discusses the responsibilities and level of performance in the areas of education, legal and ethical status, practice, continuing education, and specialized nursing practice.

NAPNES has set the standards for nursing practice of LP/VNs since 1941. The most recently revised "Standards of Practice for Licensed Practical/ Vocational Nurses" was issued in 1985. The full text of the NAPNES Standards is in Appendix E. The NAPNES Standards outline the competencies expected of the LP/VN in individual and family-centered nursing care. These Standards also discuss the moral, ethical, and legal components of practical/vocational nursing.

Job Responsibilities

The broad objective of an LP/VN education is to prepare the student to become legally qualified to work under the supervision of a medical doctor, registered nurse, osteopathic doctor, or dentist as a responsible member of a health care team, performing basic therapeutic, rehabilitative, and preventive care for anyone who needs it.

On successful completion of an LP/VN program, the new graduate is expected to be competent in a number of general areas. These competencies define the minimum expectations for graduates. The competencies were first outlined in competency statements developed by the National League for Nursing councils in the late 1970s and completed in 1979. Each state has additional nurse practice acts that further define an LP/VN's role and function in that state. In addition, some state associations of education are defining entry-level competencies.

The range of specific nursing services provided by practical nurses is extensive. It grows as the increasing sophistication and specialization of health care keeps up with discoveries in science and technology and the needs of an ever-changing population.

An LP/VN's responsibilities are set by the employer and the charge nurse or physician that the LP/VN works under. The responsibilities may change according to institution policies regarding the LP/VN's role at different patient illness levels. What an LP/VN can do for a patient may be

Table 4-1.
Beginning LP/VN Skill Inventory

Admit patients
Assist in transferring and discharging patients
Help patients with bathing
Help patients ambulate
Assist adults, children, and infants with meals
Perform range-of-motion exercises
Maintain traction
Assist in positioning patients in bed
Care for dying patients and their families
Provide skin care
Care for ostomy sites
Give enemas
Perform urinary catheterizations
Monitor oxygen therapy
Supervise coughing and deep breathing exercises
Teach and supervise postural drainage
Perform nasopharyngeal and endotracheal suctioning
Obtain specimens
Perform cardiopulmonary resuscitation
Administer compresses, sitz baths, and therapeutic baths
Measure temperature, pulse, respiration, blood pressure
Administer oral and intramuscular injections
Provide preoperative and postoperative care
Care for patients in isolation units
Assist patients in elimination needs
Assess neurological status
Document nursing care on patient records
Contribute to patient care conferences and nursing care plans
Check emergency equipment and supplies

restricted if the patient's condition worsens. The skills an LP/VN may be expected to perform are listed in Table 4-1.

Licensing

A license to practice as a licensed practical/vocational nurse is issued by the state in which the licensing examination is passed. It is the legal authorization to perform (permission to practice) the services learned in a practical/ vocational nursing program. A license is valid for life for the person it is issued to unless it is revoked or suspended. A nursing license must be renewed periodically (usually every 2 or 3 years) as required by that state's regulations.

Like all licensed professions that serve the public, practical/vocational nursing is governed by laws that protect those providing service and the safety and welfare of the people being served. Laws that govern nursing are called nurse practice acts. The nurse practice acts of each state are administered by boards called by various names, such as board of nursing, board of nurse examiners, or nurse registration. Only eight states have separate boards for registered nurses (RNs) and LP/VNs. The rest have combined boards. The majority of board members in all states are experienced RNs. In many states, boards include LP/VNs and consumers. Boards operate under the responsibility of a state agency, or they may be independently appointed by the governor. The boards operate under their own state laws but cooperate with one another.

State boards of nursing may be authorized to perform a number of duties. They may include program curricula and standards development, approval of nursing schools, license examination and renewal, and disciplinary actions such as license and approval suspension or revocation. Anyone found in violation of the state's nurse practice act is subject to investigation and prosecution by the state board.

Legal Title

The legal title granted when a person successfully passes a state LP/VN licensing examination is either *licensed practical nurse,* abbreviated LPN, or, in California and Texas, *licensed vocational nurse,* or LVN. A license entitles the holder to enter the practice of practical/vocational nursing as described by the state.

Persons holding a license have demonstrated to the issuing authority (state board) that they have the knowledge to provide the minimal safe practices required to fulfill the duties of a practical or vocational nurse in that state.

A license belongs only to the person it is issued to. It cannot be transferred to anyone else for any reason. The unqualified use of a license is subject to legal prosecution. Reporting anyone known to be practicing without a license preserves the integrity of licenses and the licensing procedure, protects the investment of license holders, and guards unknowing consumers from potentially dangerous care.

All states require practical/vocational nurses to be licensed before they can practice. Called mandatory licensing, it helps to keep unqualified persons out of the health care system. Mandatory licensing protects the public from untrained people and upholds nursing standards set by law and nursing organizations.

Licensure Qualifications

The laws governing who qualifies to be licensed as a practical/vocational nurse are set by each state, but the trend is toward uniformity in all states. Most states require that the applicant be a graduate of a state-approved practical/vocational nursing program. The director of the school of practical/vocational nursing is required to submit an application for licensure for each graduate of the school's program to the state board of nursing. The director's signature on the application indicates to the state board of nursing that the candidate for the examination has met the theoretical and clinical requirements of that school and is considered to be ready to enter the practice of practical/vocational nursing. State boards of nursing charge a licensure application fee that in most cases must be paid by the applicant.

Originally, each state had its own licensing exam. Today, however, there is one licensing examination for practical/vocational nurses in all states. This examination is developed by the National Council of State Boards of Nursing (NCSBN) and is called the National Council Licensure Examination for Practical Nurses (NCLEX-PN). The NCLEX-PN examination for licensure as a practical/vocational nurse is administered in April and October each year by the state boards of nursing. NCLEX-PN charges a scheduling fee, which is usually paid by the applicant.

One of the major goals of your practical/vocational nursing program is to prepare you to pass the licensing examination. This examination measures your knowledge of nursing practice in a number of areas and requires that you retain information you were taught during your entire educational program. Many graduates spend the time between graduation and the date of the licensing examination reviewing their textbooks and notes. Even though the examination can be taken more than once, you and your faculty will hope that you meet or exceed the minimum score for licensure on your first attempt.

The *Test Plan for the National Council Licensure Examination for Practical Nurses* is a publication developed by the NCSBN to assist practical/vocational nurses in preparing for the examination. This publication is probably available in your school library, or you can obtain a copy for a fee by writing to the NCSBN. The address can be found in Appendix F, under "Other Nursing Organizations."

Persons who take the examination are notified of the results by their state board of nursing. Everyone who meets or exceeds the minimum score is issued a license as a practical nurse in all states except California and Texas. Nurses who pass the licensing examination in California and Texas are known as licensed vocational nurses.

Licenses are issued for a period that is determined by the issuing authority. A license must be kept current. It is a violation of the nurse practice acts to continue to practice after a license has expired or been revoked. Some states require licensees to provide proof of acceptable continuing education before a license can be renewed.

State boards of nursing have the authority to issue licenses and the right to revoke or suspend them for a variety of reasons. This authority protects patients and nurses alike by eliminating those who are incompetent or unfit for practice. The standing of practical/vocational nurses is upheld when all members of the group have the same high standards.

Licensure by Endorsement

LP/VNs must be licensed by the state in which they practice. Nurses who move to or want to work in a state in which they are not licensed must apply for licensure in that state. In most cases, this process must be completed before the nurse can work in that state. You can obtain the information you need on how to apply for licensure in another state by writing to the state board of nursing in the state in which you want to work. See Appendix F for a list of addresses of the state boards of nursing.

Disciplinary Sanctions

State boards of nursing, through nursing practice laws, have the authority to suspend or revoke nursing licenses for just cause. A nursing license can be revoked or suspended when the board of nursing finds a licensee guilty of an offense. Examples of offenses include:

1. Mental incompetence
2. Conviction of a felony
3. Guilty of fraud or deceit in obtaining a license
4. Conviction of a crime involving moral turpitude or gross immorality
5. Guilty of willful neglect of a patient
6. Unfit by reason of negligence
7. Habitual use and/or chemical dependence on drugs or alcohol
8. Violations of the nurse practice laws of the state
9. Suspended or revoked license in another state

A nurse whose right to practice is being questioned must first be notified by the state board of the charges and must be given a hearing in which to enter a defense, either in person or through an attorney, before a license can be revoked or suspended.

In addition to revoking and suspending practical/vocational nursing licenses, the state board of nursing can also, for just cause, issue letters or reprimand, refuse to issue a license, refuse to renew a license, or place a licensee on probation.

Your license to practice practical/vocational nursing is a valuable document. Always conducting yourself in a manner consistent with the standards and ethics of your profession will assure you of a long and rewarding career as a licensed practical/vocational nurse.

Discussion Questions/Learning Activities

1. What is the name of the agency that approves your practical/ vocational nursing program?
2. Write to your state board of nursing and request a copy of the laws governing the practice of practical/vocational nursing. When you receive your copy, read it carefully.
3. Discuss with your classmates how the Standards published by NFLPN and/or NAPNES may affect your nursing practice.
4. How do you think you might handle a situation in which you are asked to perform nursing skills that you are not legally permitted to do?
5. How might you handle a situation in which you observe a nurse (either a registered nurse or a licensed practical/voca- tional nurse) working while obviously chemically impaired? Does your state board of nursing offer anonymous reporting of impaired nurses?
6. You have read in the local newspaper that a nurse has been convicted of child abuse. Do you inform the state board of nursing? Give the reasons for your answer.

References

American Nurses Association. Facts About Nursing. New York: The Association, 1986.

Ellis JR, Hartley CL: Nursing in Today's World: Challenges, Issues, and Trends. Philadelphia: JB Lippincott, 1988.

Fitzpatrick ML: Prologue to Professionalism. East Norwalk, CT: Appleton & Lange, 1983.

Kalisch PA, Kalisch BJ: The Advance of American Nursing. Boston: Little, Brown, 1986.

National League for Nursing: State-Approved Schools of Nursing: LPN/LVN—1986. Publication No. 19-2162. New York: The League, 1986.

National League for Nursing: Nursing Data Review 1986. Publication No. 19-2176. New York: The League, 1987.

Nursing Theory and Nursing Process

5

Objectives

When you complete this chapter, you should be able to:

Name the four concepts included in any theory of nursing.

Briefly describe one nursing theory.

Describe the five steps of the nursing process.

Describe the benefits of the nursing process.

Explain the function of NANDA.

Discuss three ways in which a nursing care plan may be developed and/or revised.

"What are you doing to my father?"

Vera looked up from her chart into the face of a very angry young man. She recognized him at once. He was the son of her patient in Room 410, Walter Simpkins. The son's name was Ray. Vera had met Ray a number of times when he was visiting his father.

Vera closed the cover on the chart she was writing and stepped outside the nurse's station. "What's the trouble, Mr. Simpkins?"

"I want an explanation, and I want it now," the man said loudly.

The RN who was Vera's team leader had left the unit for a moment. Vera, an LPN, was the only health care staff member there. She was much younger than the man, but she spoke with authority.

"I really don't know what you mean," Vera said. "Can you tell me more?"

The man calmed down. "I went to my father's room, like I do every day, to take him to the lobby, where we can talk," he said. "He told me you people are making him drink gallons of water all day long."

"I think I understand," she said. "And it isn't really gallons, Mr. Simpkins. It's more like a half a glass every 2 to 3 hours."

Ray appeared sheepish. "I—well, Dad was upset . . ."

"We know he's upset," Vera said. "But he was becoming dehydrated."

Ray nodded approval. "I'm glad to know the nursing staff is on top of things." He turned and calmly walked down the hall to his father's room.

Vera returned to her charting. "If they only knew how carefully we assess our patients," she said to herself. She opened the chart. It was filled with notations and observations. "How else could we plan what to do for our patients to help them back to health?"

What Ray and most others unfamiliar with the practice of nursing do not know is that virtually everything Vera and all nurses do is based on a broad body of knowledge and thought developed from the thinking of many professional nurses over many years of careful research and study. What may appear to a patient or a patient's relative to be random care is in reality the precise application of practices that have been thought out thoroughly, applied, and constantly revised. The practices, derived from nursing theories, are the foundation of professional nursing today.

As you learned in Chapter 3, in earlier times, nurses depended on the clergy to guide their activities. Until as recently as 30 years ago, nurses relied on other disciplines, such as medicine, to define their practice. Nurses were not encouraged to make independent decisions based on their own objectives. Today, however, nurses view nursing as a profession distinct from other professional occupations.

For any profession to advance, its educational programs and its practices must be based on a unique body of knowledge. As part of the process of becoming a separate, distinct profession, nursing has developed a body of knowledge and thought referred to as nursing theory.

A *theory* is an explanation of the nature of something. A *nursing theory* attempts to describe or explain the nature of nursing. Nursing theory guides the practice of nursing by providing a focus from which the nurse cares for other human beings.

You may hear the term "nursing model" used interchangeably with the term "nursing theory." Although there are some differences between theories and models, both attempt to describe or explain the nature of nursing. Therefore, in this book, "nursing theory" and "nursing model" are used to mean the same thing.

Beginning with Florence Nightingale, a number of nurses have developed nursing theories. Although each theory is unique, all are similar in that they explain how nursing approaches four basic concepts: the person, the environment, health, and nursing.

The major work in developing nursing theory took place in the late 1950s and early 1960s. Since then, many nursing theories have been advanced by nursing scholars. Several of these theories are summarized in Table 5-1.

An understanding of nursing theory will help you as a student and as a practitioner. A specific nursing theory or a combination of nursing theories have been used as a basis for the design of your educational program. Theory also provides the perspective from which nursing service is designed in health care facilities. By understanding how nursing theory guides your activities in nursing, you are better able to be an active partici-

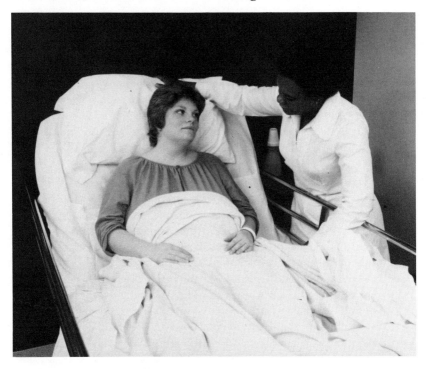

Nursing theory provides a focus from which the nurse cares for other human beings.

pant in your educational program and, in practice, a stronger contributor to the nursing team.

By studying the thinking of nursing theorists, you will begin to be able to refine your own beliefs about person, environment, health, and nursing. You will be challenged to grow in your understanding of yourself and your role as a member of the nursing team.

Nursing theories have become the guidelines of the nursing profession. There are many theories. The first was Florence Nightingale's, in 1859. Her views on nursing prevailed for almost 100 years. It was not until the early 1950s that new theories were developed. Since then, many other theories have been advanced by nursing scholars.

Nursing education programs, including yours, are based on one or more nursing theories. Nursing theory is also used to design nursing service in health care facilities. Because these two applications of nursing theory— education and service—are the foundation of your nursing career, it is important for you to have a working understanding of nursing theory.

Table 5-1.

Selected Nursing Theories and Models

Theorist	Theme	Person	Environment	Health	Nursing
Nightingale, Florence 1859	Environment affects health	Has physical, intellectual and spiritual attributes	Those aspects outside the person that affect health	Being free of disease	Putting the person in the best condition for nature to act upon him
Henderson, Virginia 1955	Principles (14) or components of nursing care	Mind and body are inseparable	Can be either a negative or positive influence on the person	Ability to function independently in the physiological environmental, and social aspects of life	Deliberate plan to meet the 14 components of nursing care
Orem, Dorothea 1958	Basic human needs are met through self-care activities	An integrated whole, with physiological, psychological, and sociological components	Created by society; includes values and expectations	Ability to meet self-care needs	Nursing education gives nurses the legitimate right to assist patients to meet self-care needs
Roy, Sister Callista 1964	Stressors affect how a person adapts	Biopsychosocial being in a changing environment	All internal and external influences that affect the human being	Health and illness are relative terms and exist at different times in differing degrees	Nurses' role to help the person adjust changes in stimuli
Neuman, Betty 1972	Systems approach to meeting human needs	An integrated whole in a constant state of change because of dynamic interrelationship of many variables	An external and an internal environment, both of which constantly affect the development of the person	Health seen as relative, depending on physiological psychological, sociocultural, and developmental state of the person	Concerned with total person and attempts to either reduce or minimize effects of external or internal stress on the person

Nightingale (1859)

Nursing care in the United States and in England was based for many years on Florence Nightingale's nursing theory. It was a framework of her ideas about what she believed nursing should be, on the basis of her observations and experiences.

Florence Nightingale believed that nursing care delivery should be based on the laws of health, which said that in the right environment, a patient would get better through natural healing processes. A nurse's duty was to provide the right environment. This was done by providing physical care and attention to the environment.

Environment was emphasized in Nightingale's time because people lived in crowded, unsanitary conditions, epidemics of disease were common, social conditions were strained, and medicine as a science was still in its infancy. There was little that could be done except to make a patient comfortable in a clean environment.

Henderson (Theory First Published in 1955)

Virginia Henderson described her theory of nursing in her book titled *The Nature of Nursing: A Definition and Its Implications, Practice, Research, and Education*, which was first published in 1955. In the second edition, which was published in 1966, she defined nursing as follows:

> The unique function of the nurse is to assist the individual, sick or well, in performance of those activities contributing to health or its recovery (or to a peaceful death) that he/she would perform unaided if he/she had the necessary strength, will or knowledge. And to do this in such a way as to help him/her gain independence as rapidly as possible [p. 15].

Henderson believes that health is basic to human functioning, and an individual's ability to function independently depends on health. She listed 14 components of basic nursing care that are intended to contribute to a patient's independence. The 14 components are as follows:

1. Breathe normally.
2. Eat and drink adequately.
3. Eliminate body waste.
4. Move and maintain a desirable position.
5. Sleep and rest.
6. Dress, undress, and select suitable clothing.
7. Maintain body temperature by adjusting clothing and environment.
8. Keep the body clean and well groomed and protect the skin.

9. Avoid changes in the environment and personal safety.
10. Communicate to express emotions, needs, fears, or opinions.
11. Worship.
12. Work to acquire a sense of accomplishment.
13. Play or participate in various forms of recreation.
14. Learn, discover, satisfy curiosity for normal development and health, and use health care facilities.
   (pp. 16-17, 1966).

Each of these 14 components of nursing care, according to Henderson, should be individualized to accommodate the uniqueness of each patient. The goal of nursing care is to assist the patient until he is able to perform these components independently.

Orem (Theory First Published in 1958)

Self-care—the things people do "on their own behalf in maintaining life, health, and well being"—is the main theme of Dorothea Orem's nursing theory. Orem sees humans as functioning biologically, symbolically, and socially, with specific needs in each of those areas. To her, health means being able to meet these needs for oneself. Orem's universal self-care requisites or needs are somewhat similar to the 14 components identified by Henderson.

When someone is unable to provide his own care, in whole or in part, the need for nursing is indicated to compensate for the deficiency and thus increase the person's ability to live to his potential in his environment. How much nursing is required is determined by the person's specific needs. Orem divides nursing intervention into three categories:

1. In *wholly compensatory nursing,* the nurse provides virtually all of the patient's self-care needs, as in intensive care and total care situations.

2. In *partly compensatory nursing,* the patient and the nurse work together to make up for the patient's limitations. As an example, the patient may be able to bathe unassisted but needs someone to change a dressing.

3. In *supportive-educative nursing,* the patient can provide self-care or could learn how to do so but needs help to learn or to adjust. Teaching a patient how to live normally within the limits of a diabetic diet is an example of this type of nursing.

In Orem's theory, the nurse has a legitimate role in helping the patient meet his self-care needs by virtue of their education specifically for this purpose.

Roy (Began Work on This Model in 1964)

Sister Callista Roy proposes that a person's ability to adapt to his environment is the basis of an effective nursing model. Her adaptation model says that people face a constantly changing environment and must adapt to it. The conflict between the changing environment and the need to adapt to it produces stress. A person's response to stress is observable behavior that combines physiological, intellectual, and behavioral reactions. How well or how poorly the person copes with stress determines how much stress is reduced or eliminated, which in turn affects health.

Health, for Roy, can be represented by a continuous line from very ill to very healthy. Successful coping with stress produces better health; unsuccessful coping produces worse health. The nurse's goal is to help the client cope so that better health can be gained. The nurse does this by first assessing the patient's needs and then intervening to see that those needs are fulfilled. This is done with the client's active participation.

Neuman (Theory First Published in 1972)

In Betty Neuman's health care systems model, the client is viewed as a whole being of many parts in an environment consisting of internal, external, and interpersonal elements. The combination is a system in which all its parts are constantly interacting. This health care model implies that to understand one thing about a person, you must take into account everything about him—not only what is happening to him, but what he is doing in response.

Forces, or stressors as Neuman calls them, act on people from inside and from outside. They may benefit or harm the individual they act on, and they can be either strong or weak. They tend to upset the individual's stability, which is the ideal condition to be in. To remain stable, the person reacts to stress by using his energy.

A person's health is defined by the amount of energy he has available to respond to stress. It is determined by comparing his normal condition with a present condition. High energy is good health. Low energy is illness. No energy is death. The person maintains good health, called stability or harmony, by using energy to balance the effects of stress.

In this model, nursing's aim is to identify stressors produced on the client by any part of the system and to intervene to reduce or eliminate them. Interventions should (1) prevent stressors from reaching the client, (2) treat stressors after they reach the client, or (3) return the client to good health after treatment.

Nursing Theory and Its Relationship to Nursing Practice

Some trends in nursing theory development can be identified, and these trends are evident in today's nursing practice. Early theorists, Florence Nightingale, for example, were more concerned with environment than with person, health, or nursing. Henderson's and Orem's models emphasize the concept of nursing as a relationship between the patient and the nurse. Neuman's health care system model emphasizes the relationship between the patient and the health care system. Physiological, psychological, socio-logical, and developmental factors are identified as some of the stressors that may have a positive or negative effect on the individual.

The trend from environment toward greater emphasis on the person in nursing theory development has led to more concern by nurses for the patient as a person. Total patient care and primary care (see Chapter 7) are intended to meet the unique needs of *individual* patients rather than groups of patients.

One of the most significant outcomes of nursing's increased interest in the uniqueness of each human is an attempt to meet the nursing and health care needs of *that* person. Who is the person? What are his or her health goals? How can nurses help the patient or client achieve these goals? These are some of the questions asked by contemporary nurses.

Madeleine Leininger, a nurse and an anthropologist, is the founder and leader in the field of transcultural nursing. Through her initial efforts in the mid-1960s, nurses began to consider the cultural differences of their patients and clients. Transcultural nursing encourages the appreciation of all cultures and discourages imposing your own cultural practices on the lives of others. This means respecting other cultures and adapting nursing care to meet the needs of people from cultures other than the nurse's. Transcultural nursing is indeed the application of those nursing theories that stress understanding the whole person in the context of their total environment. Nurses who consider the political, spiritual, economic, and cultural values of their patients before planning nursing care are practicing transcultural nursing.

The United States is made up of people from diverse cultural back-grounds. In the 1700s, people emigrated primarily from Great Britain and Germany; in the early 1800s, most immigrants were from Ireland and Ger-many; and in the late 1800s, most immigrants came from southern and eastern Europe. In the early 1900s, a large number of people came to the United States from Italy, Russia, and central European countries. Since the late 1970s and early 1980s, a large number of immigrants have come to the United States from Asia and Latin America.

Adapting to the culture and customs of the United States is often difficult, and immigrants have special needs when they require health care. Your sensitivity when caring for patients, regardless of their country of birth, can help you learn about different cultures and how to adapt your nursing knowledge and skills to the uniqueness of each patient.

Nursing Process

Translating nursing theories and models into practice is accomplished through the nursing process. The nursing process is a systematic, organized method of practicing nursing.

The nursing process consists of five steps:

1. Assessing the patient
2. Formulating the nursing diagnosis
3. Planning nursing care
4. Implementing the plan
5. Evaluating the effectiveness of nursing care

The first step, assessment, is done by observing the patient and asking questions of the patient or client or of his family or significant other. Things you can see are called objective observations; things that a patient says are called subjective reports. Objective observations include vital signs, skin condition, body language, and physical characteristics such as height and weight. Subjective reports include a patient's description of his pain, his symptoms, or his discomfort.

The second step in the nursing process is formulating the nursing diagnosis. A nursing diagnosis is a statement that describes an existing or potential health problem that nurses can treat separately from physician orders. The nursing diagnosis is made on the basis of information collected during the assessment phase or step 1 of the nursing process.

To improve communication among nurses and to assist in nursing research, an organization called the North American Nursing Diagnosis Association (NANDA) developed a standardized list of nursing diagnoses. The members of this organization discuss, review, and study research reports on proposed nursing diagnoses before including them in the NANDA-approved list of accepted nursing diagnoses. A complete list of nursing diagnoses approved for use in 1988 is found in Appendix G.

Planning, the third step in the nursing process, includes setting priorities and writing the nursing care plan. The sample nursing care plan in Table 5-2 demonstrates how a nursing care plan should look.

Table 5-2.
Sample Nursing Care Plan

Date of Admission: 8/24   **Reason for Admission:** Was involved in 2 car accident (no one else injured) and suffered ® rib fracture c̄ hemo-pneumothorax

Discharge Goal: To return to home to recuperate; to be able to do own ADL.

Age: 29   **Occupation:** Construction Worker   **Household Members:** Wife & baby girl   **Religion:** ____ Prot.

Nursing Diagnosis/ Problem	Client Outcome (Goal)	Target Date	Nursing Orders	Evaluation/ Progress

8/24
 1. Potential Fluid Volume Deficit related to fluid intake as manifested by verbalizing that he hates to drink H₂O
	Will drink at least 2000 ml daily	q shift	8/25/85
			 1. Encourage fluid intake to 2000 ml/ day as follows:
			    8ᴬ–4ᴾ = 1000 ml
			    4ᴾ–12ᴾ = 700 ml
			    12ᴬ–8ᴬ = 300 ml
			 2. Offer OJ, cranberry juice, iced tea (dislikes H₂O & milk).
			 3. Keep 7-Up at bedside.
			 4. Have him keep a record of daily fluid intake.
			            B. MacIntyre, RN
				8/25 Needs much encouragement, but does drink. BM
				
				 8/25 Keeping written record. BM

8/25 2. Potential Ineffective Airway Clearance related to pain from incisional site as manifested by a weak cough effort and statements of pain c̄ cough	Will cough and deep breathe q 2° for 2 days	q shift	8/25/85 1. Offer pain med ½° before coughing session. 2. Splint incision c̄ pillow. 3. Reinforce importance of coughing. 4. Assist c̄ coughing q 2°. B. MacIntyre, RN	8/25 Cough is still weak. Needs much encouragement. Productive of thick white mucus. BM 8/26 Improved cough effort. Cough productive as above. BM
8/26 3. Immobility related to bed rest and chest tubes as manifested by restrictive chest tubes.	Will turn and reposition himself q 2°	q shift	8/26/85 1. Assist to reposition himself q 2°—has trouble lying on ® side. 2. Reinforce the importance of moving while in bed. 3. Encourage movement of legs q 2°. B. MacIntyre, RN	8/26 Moves well c̄ assistance. BM

From Alfaro, R. *Application of Nursing Process: A Step-by-Step Guide to Care Planning.* Philadelphia, J.B. Lippincott, 1986, p. 128.

The nursing care plan is developed in several ways. One way it can be developed is by the professional nurse who admits the patient to a particular unit or service or by the primary nurse who is responsible for planning comprehensive care for a particular patient.

Another way the nursing care plan may be developed is through a formal patient care conference. The patient care conference may include only members of the nursing team, or it may be a multidisciplinary conference. A multidisciplinary conference includes nurses, social workers, physicians, pharmacists, often the family, dieticians, physical and occupational therapists, and others who are involved in providing care for a particular patient. In either case, the meeting is held to develop a plan of care based on the patient's total needs as an individual.

Yet another way a nursing care plan may be developed is less formal than the previous two methods. Nurses contribute to the care plan and revise it as the patient's condition and needs change. In this situation, the care plan is written by those nursing team members who have information relative to the condition of the patient or who become aware of nursing measures that assist the patient to achieve maximum health.

Step 4, implementation, is the step in which the care plan is put into practice. From looking at the sample care plan, you can see that specific nursing measures are prescribed for this patient. The nursing team members should implement (put into practice) the recommendations made in the

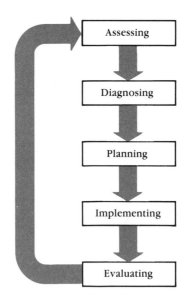

Steps of the nursing process.

nursing care plan. Problems in implementing the care plan should be reported to the professional nurse responsible for the patient unit or department.

The fifth and last step in the nursing process is the evaluation of the effectiveness of the care. It is at this point in the nursing process that the nurse evaluates how well the nursing interventions worked in assisting the patient to achieve his health goals. Evaluation of the care plan and of how it is implemented is a continuous process and often results in reassessment of the patient, revision of the nursing diagnosis, and changes in the nursing care plan.

Planning patient care by using the nursing process helps you organize your approach to the patient. It requires you to integrate your knowledge of nursing, health, person, environment, and medicine to best serve the needs of the patient. It helps you communicate with other members of the nursing team, and helps them communicate with you. Above all, the patient benefits from the quality of care that the nursing process encourages.

Discussion Questions/Learning Activities

1. Ask a nurse who graduated from nursing school 10 to 15 years ago to describe changes in nursing practice.
2. Discuss how nursing theory was used to develop your educational program.
3. What is your definition of health, and how does your definition differ from that of your classmates?
4. What are some of the ways you might handle a situation in which a patient refuses to accept nursing or health care? How will you feel?
5. Read several actual nursing care plans for patients in your clinical facility. Can you provide the rationale (reasons) for the nursing orders?

References

Alfaro R: Application of Nursing Process: A Step-by-Step Guide to Care Planning. Philadelphia, JB Lippincott, 1986.

Carpenito LJ: Handbook of Nursing Diagnosis. Philadelphia, JB Lippincott, 1987.

Fitzpatrick J, Whall A: Conceptual Models of Nursing: Analysis and Application. East Norwalk, CT, Appleton & Lange, 1983.

Henderson V: Principles and Practices of Nursing. New York, Macmillan, 1978.

Iyer PW, Taptich BJ, Bernocchi-Losey D: Nursing Process and Nursing Diagnosis. Philadelphia, WB Saunders, 1986.

Leininger M: Transcultural Nursing Concepts: Theories and Practices. New York, John Wiley, 1986.

Murray RB, Zentner JP: Nursing Concepts for Health Promotion. East Norwalk, CT, Appleton & Lange, 1985.

Neuman B: The Neuman Systems Model: Application to Nursing Education and Practice. East Norwalk, CT, Appleton & Lange, 1982.

Nightingale F: Notes on Nursing: What It Is and What It Is Not. New York, Dover Publications, 1969 (originally published in 1859).

Orem D: Nursing: Concepts of Practice. New York, McGraw-Hill, 1985.

Roy C: Introduction to Nursing: An Adaptation Model. East Norwalk, CT, Appleton & Lange, 1984.

6 The Health Care System

Objectives

When you complete this chapter, you should be able to:

Define the terms "health care provider," "health care service," "health care regulation," "health care financing," and "health care system."

Describe primary, secondary, and tertiary levels of health care.

Describe the purpose of health care regulatory agencies.

Discuss the purpose of quality assurance programs.

List the two major sources of health insurance.

Explain how DRGs are used to control the cost of health care.

Discuss the role of the U.S. government in health care.

Name the five divisions of the U.S. Department of Health and Human Services.

Outline the major functions of the Public Health Services division of DHHS.

Give three examples of current events that are increasing health care costs.

A hot shower always changed Mary Kelly's outlook on life. The shower she took one Saturday morning saved her life.

Mary was 31 years old. She was married and had a son, Erik. Her husband was a successful automobile dealer. The young family had a bright future.

As Mary lathered herself, she touched a small lump in her right breast. She had never noticed it before. She felt it again. She had two choices. She could assume the lump was not serious and do nothing, or she could make an immediate appointment with her doctor for a breast examination. For a moment Mary was undecided. Then she laughed nervously. "Oh, it's nothing," she said. She finished her shower and quickly dressed. By midmorning the lump was forgotten.

But that afternoon Mary remembered a pamphlet sent by the American Cancer Society. It told her how to do a breast self-examination. She located the pamphlet and followed its instructions. This time she immediately called her doctor.

The discovery of the lump and taking appropriate action saved Mary's life. Her own and her family's future remain secure because she knew how to use the health care system.

Obtaining health care in the United States is not often as simple as it may at first appear. Traditionally, the physician was the person who provided health care and the hospital was the place where patients went to be treated for illnesses that could not be managed in the doctor's office. Today, the health care system is far more complex, and there are many options and choices for health care. These recent changes in the health care system are sometimes confusing. This chapter will help you understand how health care is provided, regulated, and financed. Through this understanding, you will be better able to answer your patient's questions about health care, participate in approval and accreditation procedures, and contribute to reducing the costs of health care.

The Health Care System

Some general definitions will help you begin to understand the present health care system.

Health Care Providers

Health care providers are health care workers and institutions that make health care services available to those who want or need them. Physicians, dentists, optometrists, nurse practitioners, and podiatrists are examples of individual health care providers. Groups that qualify as health care providers include health maintenance organizations (HMOs) and competitive medical plans (CMPs). HMOs and CMPs charge a fee that allows clients access to all necessary medical and hospital services. This fee is not increased even for prolonged hospitalization, nor is it refunded if the client does not use any medical services.

Examples of institutional health care providers are hospitals, nursing homes, ambulatory clinics, free-standing clinics, end-stage renal dialysis clinics, and abortion clinics. Institutional health care providers provide health care services through a paid or volunteer staff, whereas individual health care providers are usually self-employed health professionals who maintain an office and see patients independently of an institution.

Individual health care providers often refer or admit patients to institutions that are also health care providers. It is important to understand that health care providers may be individuals or institutions.

Health Care Service

"Health care service" is a term used to describe the actual delivery of health care. Health care service is the diagnosis, treatment, care, and prevention of illness. It can take many forms. A surgeon who performs an appendectomy is giving health care services. The nurse who assesses a patient's vital signs is giving health care services. A dietitian who plans the week's menu for a nursing home is giving health care services. A hospital administrator who orders equipment for the physical therapy department is giving health care services. A public health nurse presenting a talk to a community group on cancer prevention is giving health care services. A volunteer in a hospice facility is giving health care services. The licensed practical/vocational nurse who is bathing a patient is giving health care service.

You will be a member of a health care team delivering health care services. Your contributions as a member of that team are vitally important to the success of the health care service.

Health Care Regulation

"Health care regulation" is a term used to describe methods designed to control not only the quality of health care but also the cost of health care. The need to regulate the quality and cost of health care can be attributed in part to the increasing complexity of society and will be discussed in more detail later in this chapter.

Health Care Financing

"Health care financing" is a term used to discuss how health care is paid for. Because health care services are costly and of national concern, this topic will be discussed in more detail later in this chapter.

Health care providers, health care services, health care financing, and health care regulation together comprise the "health care system." The goal of the health care system is to improve the health of the people in this society. There are government and nongovernment (private) components of the health care system. Government components include veterans' hospitals and nursing homes, military hospitals, and Medicare and Medicaid health insurance. Nongovernment or private components of the health care system include physicians, optometrists, dietitians, psychologists, nurse practitioners, private hospitals, nursing homes, health clinics, and private health insurance companies.

Levels of Care

Most people in the United States enter the health care system through visits to an individual health care provider because of an acute (short-term) illness or for prevention of illness. This group of health care providers is

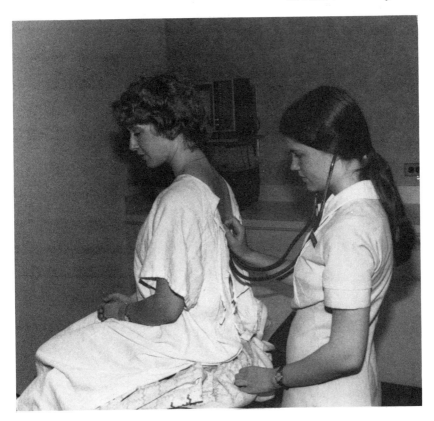

Primary level of care—the physician's office. (Courtesy of University of Michigan School of Nursing.)

called primary care providers, and the level of care they provide is called primary care.

Primary health care promotes good health and the early diagnosis and prevention of disease through services provided by physicians or nurse practitioners in offices or at ambulatory care facilities. An ambulatory care facility is one that provides health care services on an outpatient basis to limited numbers of people, usually in a limited geographic region. Examples of ambulatory care facilities include hospital clinics, free-standing medical clinics, and outpatient departments of hospitals.

Secondary health care is the diagnosis, treatment, and other care that comes after a patient enters the health care system. It is usually provided at a hospital that has specialized equipment, laboratories, and personnel. A general hospital is an example of a facility that provides secondary health care, and nurses are an example of specialized personnel.

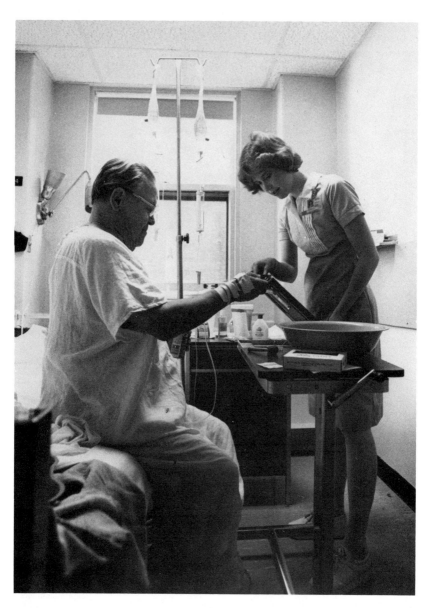

Secondary level of care—the hospital. (Photo by Bob Kalmbach, University of Michigan Information Services.)

Most secondary care is provided in institutions where a patient's admission is controlled by the institution and the physician. A patient's access to health care services is usually controlled by the attending physician (the patient's doctor). All orders for treatments, drugs, diagnostic tests, and other services must come directly from the patient's doctor or by the doctor's authority. For example, before a laboratory can perform a blood test, there must be a written order from the patient's physician. Before a nurse can administer a medication, there must be a written order from the patient's physician. Even the services of other specialists, such as psychologists and dietitians, require the attending physician's written orders. In this way, physicians are largely in control of all aspects of secondary care, just as they control primary care.

Tertiary care involves rehabilitating and restoring an individual to maximum functioning potential after an acute illness. Patients who receive tertiary care are most often those who are suffering from paralysis associated with strokes, have had spinal cord injuries, have chronic illnesses that affect the functioning of the musculoskeletal system, or are unable to care for themselves because of impaired mental functioning. Tertiary care is provided by people especially educated to meet the needs of these specific groups of patients.

Rehabilitation and restorative care can be provided at rehabilitation centers, in departments that are a part of another facility such as a physical therapy unit in a general hospital, and in long-term care facilities such as nursing homes. Tertiary care may also be provided through hospice care and home nursing care.

Hospice care tends to the unique needs of the terminally ill and their families. Hospice care is a multidisciplinary approach to helping the terminally ill patient and his family with the process of dying. Health care providers emphasize the need to adapt to the reality of impending death in a comfortable and dignified manner. Hospices or the patient's home are the usual locations for hospice care.

Home nursing care, another form of tertiary care, is nursing care provided in the patient's home. Home nursing care is most often initiated after the patient is discharged from the hospital; however, hospitalization is not a prerequisite. Although well enough to be home, the patient may not be able to meet all of his specific health care needs. The nurse visits the patient at home and provides specific health care measures and often teaches the patient or family to carry out some of the procedures for self-care. Because hospital care is very costly and also because many people prefer to be with their families during an illness, home health care is increasing in importance as a method of providing patient care.

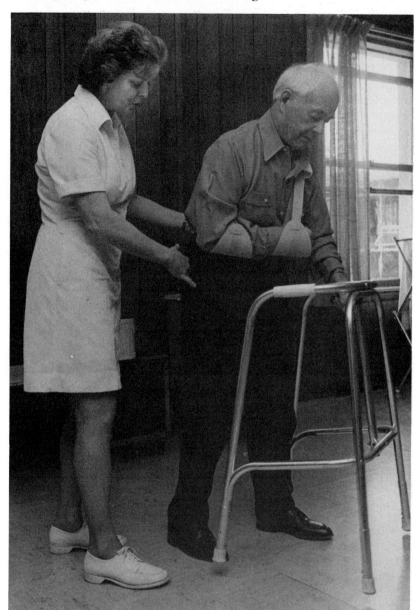

Tertiary level of care—the rehabilitation center. (Courtesy of The Jewish Home for the Aged, Portland, Maine.)

Regulation of Health Care Providers

Regulations and Primary Health Care Providers

You will recall that primary health care providers are usually those who are first to see the patient, such as a physician, a nurse practitioner, a dentist, or any one of a number of other health care providers. Primary health care providers must be licensed by the state in which they practice their profession.

Licensure is mandatory. This means that someone cannot say that he is a physician and use the initials "MD" (doctor of medicine) or "DO" (doctor of osteopathy) unless licensed to do so. And a license is usually obtained after the candidate for licensure has met educational and practice requirements and has passed a licensing examination in that particular profession.

Agencies that directly regulate the practice of primary health care providers are the licensing boards of the individual states. It is the responsibility of this board to protect the citizens of that state. Therefore the board examines applicants for licensure and issues, renews, and revokes licenses. Although licensing boards have many other responsibilities, regulating the practice of licensees is their major responsibility.

Primary health care providers are also regulated by the ethical codes of their professions. Codes of ethics will be discussed in more detail in Chapter 9.

Agencies That Regulate Hospitals

Each state department of health regulates and evaluates the activities of hospitals. To accept patients and offer medical care, hospitals must be approved by the state department of health or a similar organization. The standards affecting hospitals are applied during the evaluation process, a hospital that meets these standards is then approved to operate in that state.

Most hospitals seek accreditation from the American Hospital Association or the American Osteopathic Association. Accreditation is a voluntary process which indicates that the hospital has exceeded the minimum state standards for approval to operate a health care facility.

Agencies That Regulate Nursing Homes and Other Long-Term Care Facilities

As is the case with hospitals, nursing homes and other long-term care facilities must be approved to operate by the state department of health. In addition, nursing homes and other long-term care facilities can apply for accreditation by the American Hospital Association. In both cases, the standards for approval and for accreditation are designed to evaluate the unique health care activities that occur in these facilities. Nursing homes and long-term care facilities are not acute care hospitals; therefore the standards differ from those written for hospitals.

Regulation of Agencies That Receive Medicare and Medicaid Payments

Federal government insurance pays, through Medicare and Medicaid programs, the health care costs of a tremendous number of its citizens. To ensure that adequate services are provided at a reasonable cost, the government has established regulations that affect those hospials, nursing homes, physicians, and other providers of health care that receive reimbursement for services directly from one of these insurance plans. Many of the regulations originally established by the federal government are now being adapted for use by private insurance companies, such as Blue Cross and Blue Shield, as well as health maintenance organizations and competitive medical plans. Although many of the regulations developed by the government are very complex, they are a step toward controlling the ever-increasing cost of health care in the United States.

Quality Assurance Programs

One of the aspects of the federal regulation of health care providers who are paid for their services through Medicare or Medicaid or both is the requirement for developing quality assurance programs. Quality patient care is a goal shared by all members of the health care team, but providing that quality in a complex society with many recent technological advances is not as easy as it may seem. The purpose of quality assurance programs in health care is to evaluate and improve the level of service to patients to ensure that at least minimally accepted levels of service are provided.

Quality assurance programs generally have two major components. The first is to set standards for excellence in care. This is usually done by a committee of people who are experts in a particular area. For example, nurses who have an extensive educational background in maternity nursing and several years' experience working with women in the maternity department meet together and define, in writing, standards of nursing care that would ensure excellence.

The second step in quality assurance is to compare the actual care given against those written standards. If the actual care given does not meet the standards, changes must be made.

The Utilization and Quality Control Peer Review Organization (shortened to PRO) was created by Congress in August 1982 to ensure that health care providers who are paid by Medicare (a federal insurance program) provide care according to or above a predetermined standard. Defining standards of medical care and measuring how well health care providers meet those standards of care are far more complex than this simple explanation indicates.

Included in the PRO program is something called peer review. Peer review can be described as the examination of someone's work by other people of equal standing. In other words, physicians examine the work of other physicians, professional nurses examine the work of other professional nurses, and practical/vocational nurses examine the work of practical/vocational nurses.

Because quality assurance programs in health care facilities are becoming the rule rather than the exception, you will most likely be employed in an agency that has a quality assurance program. Your employer will expect you to provide a certain standard of care, to keep accurate written records, probably to serve on special committees, and perhaps to participate in a peer review program.

Financing Health Care

The health care system in the United States is at a critical place in its history. In 1980, more than $200 billion was spent for health care. It is projected that by the year 2000, the cost of health care will increase to more than $400 billion. Over 90% of health care costs are paid by health insurance. The two major sources of health insurance are private health insurance and government health insurance. Other sources of payment for health care are voluntary and private organizations.

Private Insurance

Private medical insurance is the kind a person buys as an individual or as a member of a group. This kind of insurance is sold by commercial insurance companies and others in the same way that life, homeowner's, and automobile insurance is sold. There are two basic kinds of private medical insurance plans: indemnity insurance and prepaid insurance.

Indemnity insurance pays its policy holder or assignee (someone authorized to receive payment, such as a health care provider) the amount stated on the policy when an approved claim is made. This amount may pay for all or a part of the claim, depending on the amount of coverage purchased. The cost of the policy will vary with the amount of coverage desired, the amount of the deductible, the insured person's age and health, and other factors. Blue Cross insurance and Blue Shield insurance are examples of indemnity insurance. Most indemnity insurance plans pay only for purchased services that result from a claim that is specifically covered in the policy. Usually the insured person may choose the care provider, as long as that provider or the services provided are not specifically excluded.

The second type of private insurance, prepaid insurance, often stresses the importance of disease prevention. These plans provide a range of prepaid services to their policyholders. The HMOs and CMPs are examples of prepaid insurance plans.

In an HMO the policyholder pays a set monthly (or other period) charge. The payment entitles the policyholder to use the plans' services for routine health care and hospitalization as needed. Some plans include long-term care and other services. The cost of the plan varies according to the services offered. The policyholder usually does not get to choose a health care provider. An HMO's primary health care providers (e.g., physicians, nurses) are usually salaried employees of the HMO or CMP or work under contract. Employee salaries are not directly related to the services provided.

There are advantages and disadvantages to each type of insurance. With indemnity insurance, the insured person can choose his provider and health services facilities. The HMO subscriber must receive treatment by the HMO member providers. On the other hand, indemnity insurance does not generally pay for preventive care, as HMOs and CMPs do. This distinction is diminishing and will probably continue to do so if studies show that preventive measures actually reduce hospitalization and the costs that accompany it.

Government Insurance

In 1965 the federal government passed legislation that made it a major health care insurance provider. The Social Security Act of 1965 included Titles XVIII and XIX, better known as Medicare and Medicaid. Medicare is a wholly federal health insurance program. Medicaid is a joint federal-state health insurance program.

Medicare is a hospital and health care insurance plan for persons 65 years of age and older. Money for this program comes from Social Security taxes paid by workers and their employers to the federal government. The services provided under Medicare are the same nationwide.

Medicaid, a state-administered program, pays for health care services for the poor of any age with funds that come from both the state and federal governments. Because Medicaid is administered by the state, the services it provides vary from state to state.

Medicare and Medicaid clients may choose their health care services and facilities from participating health care providers. Although not all health care providers accept Medicare and Medicaid patients, the majority will accept these insurance plans as payment for services. Those who do not accept Medicare and Medicaid insurance patients cite smaller payments and slow payments as reasons for not accepting these patients.

Diagnosis Related Groups

From 1965 to 1983 the Medicare program paid health care providers (e.g., physicians, hospitals, nursing homes) for services provided to people who were eligible for health care under the Medicare program. This system, called retrospective payment, meant that the health care provider ordered any and all medical care he or she believed was necessary or desirable, without consideration of the cost. The providers were reimbursed by Medicare for their costs.

As a consequence of rising health care costs, a new payment system was instituted in 1983. This system, called the prospective payment method, was developed by the federal government in an attempt to control health care costs associated with the Medicare program. The principle of prospective payment is to set rates for health care services in advance, rather than after the service has been delivered.

For example, under a prospective payment plan the cost for the treatment of appendicitis would be calculated and fixed ahead of time. The calculated cost would allow for the appropriate care of the patient and for an ordinary profit for the treating facility. If the hospital and physician delivered the treatment below the fixed rate, they would keep the difference, but if actual costs exceeded the allowable rate, they would have to bear the extra expenses themselves.

To determine the costs of treatment in advance of that treatment required a plan that the government named *diagnosis related groups* (DRGs). This is a system for classifying patients on the basis of a list of 467 medical diagnoses. Medicare patients are assigned a DRG category according to age, diagnosis, and complications. Each DRG has a set amount of money that will be paid by Medicare. By knowing the amount of reimbursement that will be received for services to Medicare patients, hospitals and other health care providers can control how much they will spend and thus ensure a profit while still providing the necessary health care.

Health Care Agencies and Organizations

Health Care and the U.S. Government

The federal government became active in health care for citizens of the United States when medical care was authorized for American merchant seamen in 1798. Since then the federal government has been involved with many health-related issues in areas of regulation, prevention, and control.

The U.S. Department of Health, Education, and Welfare was created in 1953 to address the health, education, and social concerns of Americans. This department was divided into the Department of Health and Human Services and the Department of Education in 1980.

The Department of Health and Human Services (DHHS) is divided into five divisions:

1. Office of Human Development Services (HDS)
2. Public Health Services (PHS)
3. Health Care Financing Administration (HCFA)
4. Social Security Administration (SSA)
5. Family Support Administration (FSA)

Figure 6-1 depicts the organization of the DHHS.

The Office of Human Development Services is concerned primarily with the health and welfare of elderly persons, children, youth and families, and Native Americans. Public Health Services is that division of the DHHS which is most concerned with diseases, their prevalence, and treatment; it will be discussed in more detail in the next paragraph. The Health Care Financing Administration administers Medicare and Medicaid programs. The Social Security Administration collects and disburses money under the Social Security Act. The Family Support Administration is concerned with ensuring support payments to single-parent families.

The division of the DHHS of particular interest to nursing is Public Health Services. Figure 6-1 indicates that there are six separate agencies under Public Health Services: the Centers for Disease Control (CDC), the Food and Drug Administration (FDA), the Health Resources and Services Administration (HRSA), the National Institutes of Health (NIH), the Alcohol, Drug Abuse, and Mental Health Administration, and the Agency for Toxic Substances and Diseases Registry.

The Centers for Disease Control is concerned with the prevention and control of diseases. It maintains statistics on diseases and their spread and supports research for controlling communicable diseases.

The Food and Drug Administration, through its various bureaus, protects the public from impure and unsafe foods, medications, and cosmetics;

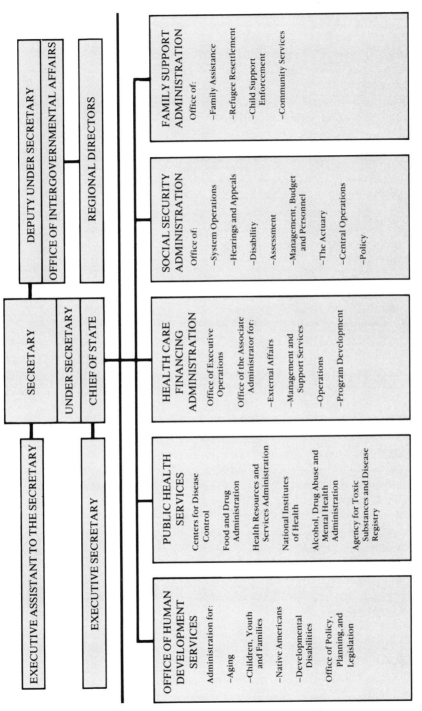

Figure 6-1. Department of Health and Human Services.

regulates the use and labeling of medicines and devices for preventing and treating diseases; sets food additive and labeling standards; conducts research; develops policy; and provides information.

The Health Resources and Services Administration emphasis is on health care resource problems in the areas of health care personnel, health care facilities, and health care delivery systems. This division is also concerned with providing leadership in planning and delivering health services.

The National Institutes of Health comprises over a dozen separate agencies. The National Cancer Institute, the National Institute of General Medical Sciences, the National Institute on Aging, and the National Institute on Nursing are examples. Each agency is engaged in the research and treatment of specific problems.

The Alcohol, Drug Abuse, and Mental Health Administration directs its energies to research and treatment of health problems associated with drug and alcohol abuse and to the improvement of mental health through separate institutes.

The Agency for Toxic Substances and Diseases Registry is a recently created branch of the Public Health Service. Its mission is to assess the prevalence and effects of environmental pollutants on the health of people in this country.

All the divisions of the Public Health Service routinely share information with other countries. Although the health of Americans is the primary concern, communicable diseases, toxic waste, and diseases such as AIDS are international problems that are of concern to the Public Health Service.

State and Local Health Departments

State governments also have agencies that regulate and oversee the delivery of health care services. A commissioner of health, a secretary of health, or someone with a similar title is assigned the responsibility of overseeing health programs in his particular state. This office also administers the state Medicaid health insurance program for residents with low income.

State health department functions may also include the licensing of health care workers, hospitals, nursing homes, pharmaceutical manufacturers and distributors, and other health care agencies. State health departments also disseminate information and educational material such as films, books, and pamphlets on health matters to both the general public and health care agencies.

Divisions of the state health department may include public health, communicable diseases, vital statistics, maternal and child health, mental health, and other programs. The state health department in some areas has a direct relationship with local health departments.

Local health departments place their emphasis on the health care needs of people living in specific geographic areas. Their jurisdiction may include a town, a city, a county, a borough, or some other clearly defined area. Functions of the local health department include reporting communicable diseases, keeping vital statistics, managing sanitation, providing a safe water supply, providing child and school health services, and managing other matters of local public health.

Private Organizations That Support
Health Care Services

The health care system in the United States also includes a large assortment of private organizations dedicated to meeting specific health care needs of the population. National organizations include the American Heart Association, the American Cancer Society, the March of Dimes Birth Defects Foundation, the United Way, and many, many more. Financial support for these organizations comes from fund drives, individual contributions, business and corporate gifts, and donations. Although these organizations do not generally provide health care, they do contribute millions of dollars to support research and treatment of specific diseases.

Private funding for health care services also includes community drives that raise money to help an identified individual or family cope with a catastrophic and expensive illness. You have probably been approached by a friend or neighbor and asked to contribute to a health care fund for a needy individual in your community. These people-to-people programs do a great deal to improve the health of this society.

The private organizations contribute millions of dollars that would otherwise not be available to conduct research and to treat patients who have some of the more common diseases in this country. Their contribution to the health care system must be recognized, supported, and appreciated by everyone.

Future Concerns

In spite of efforts by the federal government to reduce spending for health care, costs are continuing to increase. There are several reasons why this trend is difficult to change. One of the most significant reasons for this increase in health care costs is the increase in the number of elderly people in America. In 1985 there were 28.5 million people age 65 years and older. By the year 2000, that number will increase to about 35 million, and by the year 2025, it is expected that 58.6 million people will be at least 65 years of age. Increasing age does not necessarily mean illness, but many older people do have extensive and expensive health care needs.

Another factor that will increase the cost of health care is the increase in the number of people with acquired immune deficiency syndrome (AIDS). Patients who have AIDS generally require medical care for long periods. As the incidence of the disease increases, so too does the cost of caring for these patients.

A third factor that will significantly affect the cost of health care is the critical nursing shortage. As the supply of nurses dwindles, salaries will increase and directly affect the cost of health care.

You will be in a position both to affect, and to be affected by, changes in the health care system. As the number of professional and nonprofessional nurses declines, you can expect salaries to increase. Bonuses, tuition reimbursement, and other incentives will be offered by employers.

You will affect the health care system by the efficiency with which you provide care. The goal of health care services in the future will be to provide safe, efficient, and effective care and to restore health in the shortest possible time.

Discussion Questions/Learning Activities

1. List as many different places as you can where health care providers offer health care services. (You might use the telephone directory for additional information.)

2. How is the practice of primary health care providers (physicians, nurse practitioners, and hospitals) regulated in your state?

3. Ask the librarian to direct you to the American Hospital Association or Medicare guidelines for accreditation. Briefly scan one of these documents to determine what a regulatory agency expects from an institutional health care provider.

4. Try a short peer review after your next clinical day. Ask one of your classmates to evaluate your performance during the day. How does your classmate's assessment of your performance compare with yours?

5. Ask some of your family, friends, or relatives to describe their health care insurance. Do they know what services are excluded? How much does their insurance cost, and does their employer pay any part of the cost?

(Continued)

6.   Discuss the DRG method of payment for health care with your classmates. What are the advantages and disadvantages of this system to both the patient and the health care provider?

7.   List some of the ways you can directly contribute to controlling health care costs, both as a nurse and as a consumer of health care.

References

Antrobus M: District Nursing: The Nurse, the Patients, and the Work. Winchester, MA, Faber & Faber, 1985.

Blues A, Zerwekh J: Hospice and Palliative Nursing Care. New York, Grune & Stratton, 1983.

DeBella S, Martin L, Siddall S: Nurses' Role in Health Care Planning. East Norwalk, CT, Appleton & Lange, 1987.

Hawkins JW, Hayes ER, Abner CS: An Orientation to Hospitals and Community Agencies. New York, Springer Verlag, 1986.

Hawkins JB, Higgins LP: Nursing and the American Health Care Delivery System. Tireasias Press, 1985.

Holle ML, Blatchley ME: Introduction to Leadership and Management in Nursing. Boston, Jones & Publishers, 1987.

Jonas S: Health Care Delivery in the United States. New York, Springer Verlag, 1986.

Luft HS: Health maintenance organizations: Implications for nursing. In Aiken LH (ed): Nursing in the 1980s: Crisis, Opportunities, Challenges. pp. 317–27. Philadelphia, JB Lippincott, 1982.

Roemer MI: An Introduction to the U.S. Health Care System. New York, Springer Verlag, 1986.

7

Today's Health Care Facilities and the Patient Care Team

Objectives

When you complete this chapter, you should be able to:

List the four ways in which hospitals are classified.

Compile a list and describe the function of several health care team facilities other than hospitals.

Define the term "level of care" in relation to patient units and give examples of each.

Define the term "patient care team" and describe the educational preparation of several of its members.

List the members of the nursing team and describe their major responsibilities related to patient care.

Explain and describe differences in case, functional, team, and primary nursing care delivery models.

Alice parked her car in the lot behind Riverview, the nursing home where her grandmother lived, and hurried inside.

As she approached her grandmother's room, she saw her sister, Jeanne, in the doorway. "They're taking Grandma to the hospital," Jeanne said in a worried voice. "She's having trouble breathing."

The two women accompanied the stretcher to the waiting ambulance. The old woman's breathing was labored. Alice spoke to the attendant as the stretcher was put into the ambulance. "I'm a licensed practical nurse," she said. "May I go along?"

"Sure, get in," the attendant said.

The ambulance delivered Alice's grandmother directly to the emergency department of the hospital. Alice was soon joined by her sister, who had followed in her car. "What's going to happen?" Jeanne asked. She was clearly worried.

"Don't worry," Alice said reassuringly, as she patted Jeanne's shoulder. "Grandma will get the best of care here."

The two women went to the admitting office, where a clerk took the necessary information about their grandmother. Then they returned to the emergency department.

"How is my grandmother?" Alice asked one of the nurses on duty.

The nurse smiled. "They took her up to an adult care unit. It's her heart. The doctor wants to watch her until her EKG settles down."

Alice and Jeanne went upstairs. The head nurse was speaking with the woman's physician. A lab technician stopped at the nurse's station. He spoke briefly with the unit clerk, who gave him a tray of freshly drawn blood samples. As they spoke, an orderly appeared. He handed a package from the hospital pharmacy to the clerk, who read its label and made a notation on a chart. The doctor departed.

An LPN emerged from a room down the hall and quickly disappeared into an elevator. A nurse's aide, laden with an armload of fresh bed linen, hurried by. Other RNs and LPNs moved through the halls, each with a task to do.

Jeanne watched all the activity in amazement. "Is it like this every day?" she asked.

Alice shook her head. "No," she said. "Some days it gets busy!"

A week later the sisters met again at the hospital. This time they were taking their grandmother home. Not to Riverview, but to Alice's home. A home care plan had been arranged through the hospital's social service department.

"Is this something special they did because you're a licensed practical nurse?" Jeanne asked, as Alice poured tea for her sister and their grandmother.

Alice smiled. "No. It's all a part of a team effort that works inside the health care system," she said. She winked at her grandmother, who lay propped up on a rose-colored pillow in bed, and said, "And I'm proud to be a member of the patient care team."

Until the early part of the 1900s, the traditional "health care facility" for treating illness, injury, and dying was the patient's home. The health care "team" was the patient's family. If a patient could afford the services of a physician, these services were also provided in the patient's home.

The changes in hospitals and nursing begun by Florence Nightingale during the Crimean War (1854–1856) and by American reformers after the Civil War (1861–1865) started the trend toward improvement of facilities and care that is still going on today.

Inventions such as rubber gloves, hypodermic syringes, and thermometers, scientific discoveries such as the bacterial causes of infection, and the movement of people into crowded cities added to the changing nature of health care.

Today, hospitals are the major class of health care facility, and skilled teams of professional and technical workers deliver health care to patients in every category of need.

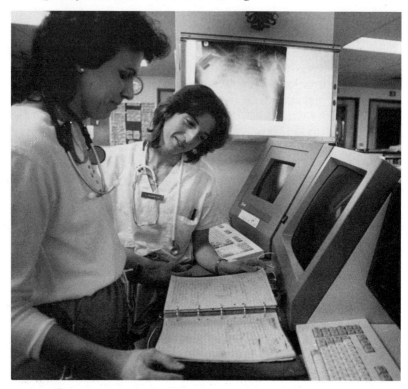

In today's hospital, technology assists skilled teams to provide patient care. (© Cliff Moore, Taurus Photos.)

Hospitals

A hospital's primary role is to provide health care. In addition, hospitals are often medical education centers. They furnish training, seminars, and resources to physicians, nurses, technicians, social workers, dietitians, therapists, emergency medical personnel, and other health and medical care specialists. Some areas of education available at hospitals include disease prevention and treatment, health maintenance, pathological analysis, and rehabilitation. Hospitals also have clinics and laboratories for the treatment, analysis, and research of illness and injury.

There are approximately 7000 hospitals in the United States. They are classified by ownership, the kind of services they offer, their size, and the length of patient stay.

Ownership can be *public* or *private*. Public hospitals are those owned by federal, state, or local governments. Veterans Administration hospitals, U.S. Public Health Service hospitals, and military hospitals are examples of hospitals owned by the federal government. State university hospitals, state mental institutions, and state prison hospitals are examples of state-owned hospitals. County and municipal hospitals are owned by local governments.

Private hospitals—also called voluntary hospitals—are owned and operated by individuals, partnerships, corporations, religious groups, and labor unions.

Hospital operated as businesses are called proprietary, investor-owned, or for-profit hospitals. Hospitals operated as services and not for profit are called nonprofit, nonproprietary, official, or not-for-profit hospitals. Public hospitals are not-for-profit hospitals. Private hospitals can be for-profit or not-for-profit hospitals, depending on their financial purpose.

Hospitals can provide general or special services. General hospitals provide health care for most kinds of disorders to patients of most ages. Most hospitals are general hospitals.

Specialty hospitals provide health care only for specific disorders or conditions or for limited age groups. Psychiatric hospitals, children's hospitals, and maternity hospitals are examples of specialty hospitals.

Teaching and research services are generally provided at larger hospitals, usually in conjunction with patient care.

Hospitals provide care for acute conditions or chronic conditions. Some facilities may provide both types of care.

Short-term care facilities provide treatment for acute conditions requiring specialized personnel and sophisticated equipment and procedures for a short time. A general hospital provides acute care.

Long-term care facilities provide treatment, maintenance, and rehabilitation for patients with chronic conditions needing extended care.

Hospitals can also be classified by the total number of patient beds available. A hospital may have fewer than 25 beds or more than 500 beds.

Hospitals can be categorized by the average length of stay of its patients. Short-term hospitals serve patients whose average stays are generally less than 30 days. Long-term hospitals care for those with average stays of 30 or more days. There are many more short-term than long-term hospitals. Again, many hospitals provide both short-term and long-term care within their facility.

"Inpatient" and "outpatient" describe patients and health care facilities according to the length of patient stay, specifically whether patients spend at least one night at the facility.

An inpatient is a patient who is admitted to a health care facility for

24-hour care. An outpatient is a patient who is treated and released from the facility without an overnight stay. Outpatients are often treated in clinics, doctor's offices, and the emergency department, all of which are a part of the usual hospital complex.

Patient Care Units and Levels of Care

Specialization in health care delivery requires specialized health care facilities. Some facilities provide a single kind of care. A nursing home, for example, specializes in long-term care for patients who, in general, require similar treatment. The range of services in a nursing home is complete for the normal needs of its clients but is limited to those needs. A nursing home would not have a surgical department or an emergency department.

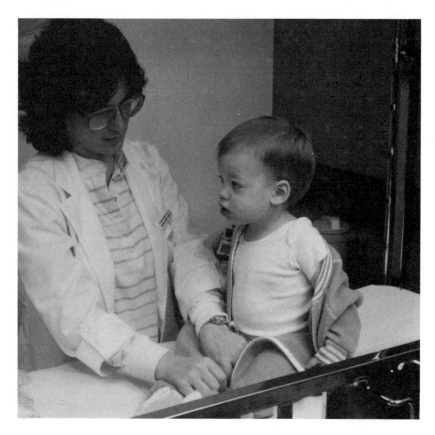

A pediatric unit specializes in caring for children.

On the other hand, a general hospital serves a wide variety of patients with an extensive assortment of services. Those services may include an emergency department, comprehensive surgical procedures, obstetrics, x-ray examinations, pediatrics, psychiatric care, and many others. Such diversity requires that each service be separated from the others for efficient management, so that services will not be duplicated and personnel will be used to the best advantage.

Patient care units that vary in size from 10 to 60 beds can be separated by the type of care provided and by the level of care required by the patient.

Units that specialize in specific types of care include coronary care, pediatric, obstetric, and psychiatric units. Depending on the size of the facility, these units may fill a portion of a floor, a whole floor, or even a wing.

Levels of patient care—how much care an individual patient needs— also can be managed in units in which all the patients in the unit require the same relative amount of care. The overall management of patients by level of care is called progressive patient care. Progressive patient care units include intensive care units and intermediate, self-care, and long-term care.

Intensive Care Units

Intensive care units are reserved for patients who are seriously or critically ill and who require total care and monitoring by means of specialized techniques and knowledge—and with the use of equipment that is immediately available in the unit. Health services personnel working in these units are highly skilled in using all available resources to assist the patient to recover from serious injury or disease or major surgery.

There are several types of intensive care units:

1. Coronary care unit
2. Surgical intensive care unit
3. Medical intensive care unit
4. Neonatal intensive care unit
5. Pediatric intensive care unit
6. Burn intensive care unit
7. Postanesthesia and recovery unit

Intermediate Care Units

Intermediate care units include the general medical and surgical units, the pediatric unit, the maternity unit, the newborn nursery, and the psychiatric unit; they are found in a general short-term ("acute") care hospital. Patients in these units are admitted for diagnosis or treatment of illness that cannot be treated on an outpatient basis. Patients admitted to these units are not critically ill; however, they do need the specialized medical and nursing care available in a hospital. Rehabilitation, including teaching patients how to care for their own health, is an important activity in intermediate care units.

Self-Care Units

Self-care units are for patients with no or minimal limits on what they can do for themselves but who still need rehabilitation and health care teaching or specialized therapy. These units are as homelike as possible. Patients eat in dining rooms, wear their own clothes, use recreational facilities, and keep their own appointments at other departments within the hospital.

Long-Term Care Units

Some short-term care hospitals have designated certain wings or floors as long-term care units. The patients in the units have needs similar to those of patients who are admitted to nursing homes. Long-term care is that care provided to patients who have an illness that may not be curable but whose condition may be improved through medical and nursing care.

Other Health Care Facilities

Other types of health care facilities that provide health services include nursing homes, rehabilitation centers, freestanding surgical centers ("surgi-centers"), end-stage renal dialysis units, doctor's offices, neighborhood health centers, local health departments, industrial health centers, and community health centers.

A nursing home is a facility that provides care, generally, to older people who cannot care for themselves. Nursing homes are classified as either skilled nursing facilities (SNFs) or intermediate care facilities (ICFs). SNFs provide skilled nursing services to patients who usually plan to return to their home. The patients in an SNF are too well to remain in a short-term care hospital but too ill to return to their home. Rehabilitation services are often an important part of an SNF. Patients in an SNF often require the level of nursing service that is directed by registered nurses and licensed practical/vocational nurses.

ICFs are designed to provide long-term care, usually to people over the age of 65 years who cannot continue to live alone or with their families. Residents of ICFs often have chronic medical problems such as senility, Alzheimer's disease, paralysis resulting from a stroke, or a generalized weakness that makes it difficult for them to care for themselves or for their families to care for them.

Rehabilitation centers may be a division within a short-term care hospital, or they may be privately owned by physicians, physical therapists, or occupational therapists. These centers work with individual patients and their families to assist the patient to achieve his maximum physical and mental potential.

Surgical centers ("surgi-centers") are a relatively new concept in health care facilities. These centers, usually not part of a hospital, provide minor surgical services for outpatients. The cost of procedures performed in these centers is less expensive than the same procedure performed in the hospital. Patients go home the same day as the surgery.

End-stage renal dialysis centers are often privately owned by physicians or other health care providers. They provide dialysis services to patients whose kidney function is inadequate. Patients report to the dialysis center three times a week for renal dialysis. The cost of renal dialysis is often covered through one of the federal government health insurance programs.

Doctors' offices can also be considered health care facilities. The major portion of health care is provided through them. There are many arrangements of doctors' offices. Some have only one doctor, whereas others have many doctors in the same facility. When several doctors share the same facility, the term "group practice" is used to describe the office.

Neighborhood health centers are usually found in low-income neighborhoods. They provide a range of health care services to people of all ages who cannot afford private medical care. These centers depend on local, state, and federal funding to subsidize the cost of the medical care they provide.

Local health departments are also health care facilities. Larger cities are often divided into health districts, with each district served by an office that provides health care to residents of that particular district. In less populated areas, the county health department may provide the same services.

Industrial health centers are facilities found in businesses and industrial plants. These centers are staffed by a variety of health services personnel. Larger businesses and industries may employ physicians and nurses and offer a broad range of diagnostic services for their employees. Some of the health centers in larger businesses and industries offer fitness centers, counseling, and other health services.

Community mental health centers are generally organized as outpatient facilities for the diagnosis and treatment of mental and emotional disorders. These centers provide counseling services for patients who can continue to live in society but are in need of specialized treatment.

Miscellaneous Services

There are many types of miscellaneous health care-related services that are provided in a variety of facilities. Although these services are not the typical ones we think of when we think of health care and health care facilities, they do contribute to the well-being of our society. These services indirectly influence health. Some of them include adult and child day care centers, Meals on Wheels, suicide and child abuse hotlines, family planning services, homemaker services, and specialized transportation services for ill and disabled persons.

In addition, many groups are organized to provide emotional and psychological support for individual and families with problems that are health related. A few examples include Alcoholics Anonymous, Women Organized Against Rape, Women Against Abuse, Reach for Recovery (for patients recovering from mastectomies), Sudden Infant Death Syndrome Foundation, and the Zipper Club (for patients recovering from heart surgery).

The Patient Care Team

All health care facilities, regardless of type, size, sophistication, or service, depend on the people who staff them for health care delivery. The biggest, best-equipped hospital is no better than the team that runs it and delivers care there, because health care comes from people, not from the tools and technology they use to provide it.

The term "patient care team" refers to all personnel in all departments associated with the delivery of medical and health care, including the administrative operations.

When you enter practice, the area of health care you choose will determine the type of facility you work in, and the type and size of the facility will determine how large and how varied a health care team it will have.

The staff of a health care facility can be large or surprisingly small, depending on the type and size of the facility itself. A major institution will have a complete health care team that would include most if not all of the team members described on pp. 125-128.

The number of departments in a health care facility can range from very many to very few. They include, among others, administrative, medical, nursing, medical records, social services, therapy, dietary, laboratory, and maintenance services.

A hospital's primary function is to deliver health care to its patients. The patient is at the center of a group of people dedicated to that objective. This group is the health care team.

Every institution has its own specific organization. Most will include variations of the following.

A health care institution's administration gets its authority from a board of directors or board of trustees. The board members are a group of responsible individuals who do not have day-to-day involvement with the facility's operation but who set its overall objectives and see that they are carried out. A board of directors has ultimate control of a facility.

Administration can be divided into two general areas: business operations and medical operations. Each area has a separate daily agenda, and each is headed by its own administrator. Both departments are accountable to the facility's chief administrator, who is called a superintendent or director. The chief administrator is accountable for the facility's overall operation to the board of directors.

Business operations are under the direction of a business manager, or comptroller. The comptroller oversees departments that manage payroll, purchasing, maintenance, and other areas of operation involving finances.

Medical operations are under the direction of a medical director (or a group of staff physicians). The medical director oversees all levels of professional care. The heads of each medical department are accountable to the medical director. Departments include, among others, the medical staff and the nursing staff, as well as nonmedical departments such as medical records, social services, physical therapy department, pharmacy, and laboratories. Some institutions have a separate nursing department with a director of nursing at its head.

Figure 7-1 shows how the administration of a typical hospital is organized.

Members of the Patient Care Team

A patient care team at a typical facility might include the following (keep in mind that advances in technology continually generate the need for skilled personnel and new job descriptions to fit them:

Administrator—a physician, nurse, or college graduate with a degree in business or hospital administration. This person is appointed by the board of trustees to oversee all hospital operations.

Dentist (DDS)—a state-licensed practitioner of dentistry with a 4-year undergraduate degree plus 4 years of dental school. Dentistry is the treatment and prevention of disorders and diseases of the teeth and related structures of the mouth, including repair, replacement, and restoration of teeth.

Dietitian—a 4-year college graduate specialist in dietetics. Dietetics involves food, nutrition, and diet planning and preparation according to sound

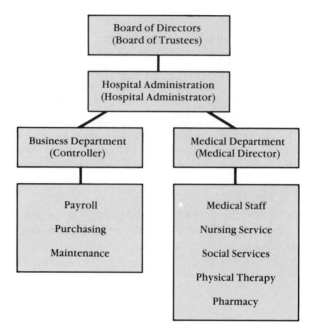

Figure 7-1. Typical organization of a hospital.

nutritional principles, especially as they relate to health and disease. A registered dietitian has passed the American Dietetic Association examination and is required to continue related education.

Electrocardiograph Technician—one who is trained on the job in the use of an electrocardiograph (EKG), a device used to record heart muscle activity to detect cardiac (heart) problems or to monitor the heart activity of patients known to have cardiac problems.

Laboratory Assistant—one trained to perform simple laboratory tests and procedures; usually a high school graduate. Specialties for laboratory technicians and technologists may require a college degree and, in some states, certification and licensure.

Licensed Practical/Vocational Nurse—a state-licensed graduate of an approved LP/VN program lasting approximately 1 year.

Medical Doctor (MD)—a physician, most often a medical or surgical specialist. An MD first completes 4 years of college and then attends an approved medical school for 4 years. After a hospital internship of 1 year and a hospital residency of up to 5 years, and after successfully passing a state licensing examination, the MD can enter practice. A general practitioner (GP) is a nonspecialist, commonly a "family doctor," who provides general health care.

Medical Technologist (MT-ASCP)—one trained and certified to work in a medical laboratory under a pathologist's supervision. A medical technologist has a minimum of 4 years of college education plus a year of training approved by the American Medical Association (AMA). MTs are certified by the Registry of Medical Technologists of the American Society of Clinical Pathologists (ASCP) on successful passing the required exam.

Occupational Therapist—one who has a minimum of 4 years of college education and helps patient readapt to daily life after illness or injury.

Optometrist (OD)—a graduate and licensed specialist in eye examination and prescribing and fitting eyeglasses.

Osteopathic Physician, Osteopathic Surgeon (DO)—a physician trained and licensed in osteopathy, a practice of medicine that emphasizes the role of the body's organs, muscles, and skeletal system in treating disease.

Pathologist—a licensed physician who specializes in the nature and causes of disease.

Pharmacist—a graduate (5 or 6 years of college, with a bachelor of science [BS] degree), licensed, and registered specialist in compounding and dispensing medications.

Physical Therapist—one who has a minimum of 4 years of college education and works with patients to regain full physical function, through exercise, massage, and other techniques, after illness or injury.

Physician's Assistant (PA)—one who is specially trained to provide assistance to a physician under the physician's direction and supervision; also called physician's associate, medex, or medic. Most PAs practice primary health care.

Podiatrist (DSC, PODD)—a graduate (usually 6 years of college), licensed specialist in the treatment of disorders of the foot.

Psychologist—a graduate (master's or doctoral degree) specialist in diagnosis, treatment, and counseling of patients with mental, emotional, or emotionally caused physical problems.

Radiologic Technologist (RT)—one trained to use x-ray equipment, fluoroscopy, radiation therapy, and the administration of radioisotopes.

Registered Nurse (RN)—a graduate, state-licensed specialist in nursing care. RNs receive their education through either diploma, associate-degree, or baccalaureate programs, after which they are qualified to take the licensing exam to become a registered nurse.

Respiratory Therapist—a graduate of 2-, 3-, or 4-year approved program that provides training in the use of gases, drugs, and equipment under medical supervision to restore normal cardiopulmonary function in patients recovering from illness or injury.

Social Worker—one who has a minimum of 6 years of college education and helps patients and their families adjust to personal problems.

A variety of other positions fill out the staff of a large health care facility. The support staff members include nursing department employees such as unit clerks and managers. Other support staff include clerical and secretarial workers, maintenance personnel, kitchen and dietary staff members, and numerous others engaged in the provision of direct and indirect services to patients.

Unit clerks, sometimes called ward clerks, work under the supervision of the head nurse or a unit manager. Their duty is to manage the clerical work at a nursing station.

A floor or unit manager is in charge of the clerical management of a whole nursing floor or unit and is under the supervision of a hospital administrator.

The management, or administrative, staff includes accountants, attorneys, human resources managers, and others whose jobs relate to the overall operation of the facility.

The Nursing Team

A nursing team may have many or few members. How closely they work together may be well defined or imprecise. The members of a nursing team may vary from institution to institution. They include RNs, LP/VNs, and student nurses, and they may also include nurse practitioners, nursing assistants, and unit managers and clerks. Others who work in conjunction with the nursing team are nurse's aides, orderlies, attendants, and various office and clerical personnel.

A nursing team operates under distinct lines of authority. Team members with higher authority—a team leader or charge nurse, for example —are responsible for directing those working under their authority. Team members working under a team leader are obligated to follow directions given by the person in charge.

Each member of a team is responsible for his own performance. It is each member's personal obligation to do the assigned work at or above the standards expected from health care workers at his level of authority and competence. Authority should not be confused with competence. A job title or assignment that gives someone the authority to perform a specific task does not qualify that person to do it. On the other hand, someone with the required skill to do a procedure does not automatically have the authority to do it. Because you are personally responsible for what you do at all times, for your own protection and the protection of your patient and employer, act only under those with authority and never act beyond the competence for which you are licensed.

Nursing team organization also will vary from facility to facility. It will be your responsibility to learn the organization of the nursing department where you are employed and to conform to the lines of authority and responsibility it sets. An example of the organization of a nursing department is shown in Figure 7-2.

A typical hospital nursing department may be headed by a director of nursing who is in charge of all nursing services.

Under the director of nursing are clinical coordinators who administer nursing services for specific programs and clinical departments, such as the nursing services used for maternal and child health care, medical and surgical service, intensive care units, or educational services for patients or certain employees. Clinical coordinators are accountable for their own departments and answer to the director of nursing. Clinical coordinators are also referred to as patient care coordinators, patient care managers, and supervisors. Regardless of the title, they are responsible for managing budget, staff, and other services necessary to operate more than one patient care unit.

Head nurses generally have the responsibility for administering the nursing care in a single patient care unit, such as the emergency department, the recovery room, or the surgical unit. They are responsible for the planning and supervision of nursing care in their units and answer to their clinical coordinator. In large nursing units, assistant head nurses or charge nurses may assume some of the responsibilities of the head nurse.

In addition to the clinical coordinator and the head nurse, the nursing team generally has the following members: staff nurses, LP/VNs, student nurses, and nursing assistants.

Staff Nurses

Staff nurses are registered nurses (RNs) who usually have direct responsibility for patient care. Typical functions of a staff nurse include assessing a patient's physical and psychological condition, administering medications, monitoring vital signs, providing personal hygiene, teaching patients and families, and carrying out treatment regimens. In addition, staff nurses develop nursing care plans based on nursing diagnoses and collaborate with physicians to resolve medical problems. Staff nurses collaborate with their head nurse and clinical coordinator to solve nursing problems.

The staff nurse is a patient advocate and, as such, communicates with other hospital departments to meet the many needs of a person receiving services in the health care system.

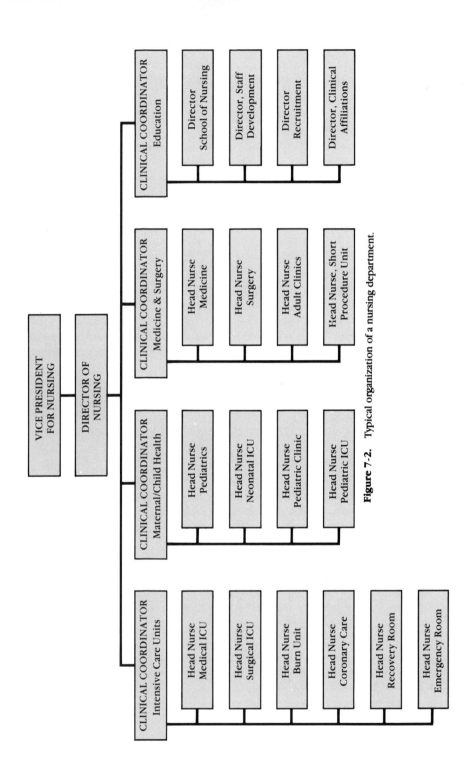

Figure 7-2. Typical organization of a nursing department.

Licensed Practical/Vocational Nurses

Under the supervision of appropriate nursing authority, LP/VNs provide nursing services for which they are licensed and qualified. The nursing authority is clearly defined in the nurse practice acts of the state in which each practical/vocational nurse works. Many state nurse practice acts require that LP/VNs work under the direct supervision of a licensed physician, registered nurse, or dentist.

LP/VNs working as a member of the nursing team are expected to be a contributing member of the team. Providing direct patient care and assisting the registered nurse in meeting the needs of the patients in a particular health care facility requires excellent communication and observation skills. The functions of the LP/VN were discussed in some detail in Chapter 4.

Student Nurses

Student nurses, whether in a registered nursing education program or in a practical/vocational nursing education program, practice clinical skills and learn under the supervision of a clinical instructor. The clinical instructor, in turn, works closely with the head nurse and other members of the

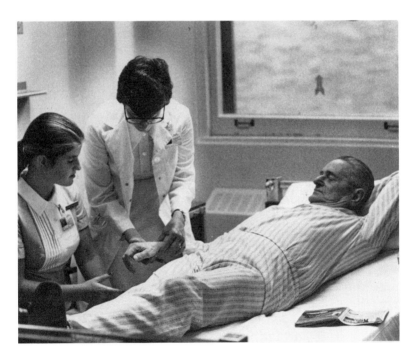

Your instructor supervises your clinical practice. (Photo by Bob Kalmbach, University of Michigan School of Nursing.)

nursing team. Clinical instructors are legally responsible for the actions of their students and, for this reason, are very careful to observe and evaluate student performance.

Student nurses do not replace staff nurses and LP/VNs on the nursing team, but they are a part of that team. As a part of that team, student nurses are expected to provide safe and competent patient care. Student nurses are expected to seek the assistance of their clinical instructor when questions regarding patient care arise.

Nursing Assistants

Nursing assistants, as members of the nursing team, help RNs and LP/VNs by providing basic nursing care to patients. Nursing assistants may also be called aides, orderlies, or attendants. Their functions generally include making beds; assessing temperatures, pulses, respirations, and blood pressures; filling water carafes; distributing and collecting meal trays; and feeding some patients.

Although the level of performance of nursing assistants may not be as sophisticated as that of some other members of the nursing team, their contributions are equally important to the success of the nursing team.

Nursing Care Delivery Methods

Methods of providing nursing care can be divided into a number of different types, or methods, to ensure the highest level of care performed in the most efficient and economical manner. The method used by one facility may differ from that of another. The decision of which method of nursing care an institution will use is made on the basis of the availability of staff and equipment, the size and nature of the physical plant, and the administrative and nursing philosophies.

As a student and later when you enter practice, you will most likely be assigned to a unit where one of the following general nursing care delivery methods is followed:

1. Case method
2. Functional nursing
3. Team nursing
4. Primary nursing

Case Method

The case method is the oldest approach to the delivery of nursing care. In this method, the nurse is responsible for the entire care of one or more patients for one shift in a 24-hour period. This method is frequently used in intensive care units and is always used in private duty nursing. It is often the method used with student nurses during their clinical experience.

Functional Nursing

Functional nursing is a system in which each nursing team member is assigned a specific function or task. For example, one team member takes the temperature of all the patients on the unit, other team members make all the beds, and so forth. Functional nursing is sometimes efficient, but it is a very fragmented approach to patient care. Patients often have a difficult time establishing a relationship with the nursing team because so many members of the team are responsible for their care.

Team Nursing

Team nursing, instituted in the mid-1950s, was intended to minimize the fragmented case associated with the functional nursing method of patient care. The team consists of a team leader, who is usually a registered nurse, staff nurses, LP/VNs, and auxiliary personnel (such as aides and orderlies). A patient unit may have two or more teams, each having responsibility for the nursing care of 10 or more patients. The team members work together to combine their diverse educational preparation to benefit their group of patients. Team conferences are held to develop individual patient care plans.

Primary Nursing

The most recently developed nursing care method is called primary care. In primary nursing, a registered nurse has total responsibility for a particular patient 24 hours a day, 7 days a week, for the entire time the patient is in the hospital. The purpose of this model is to provide continuity of care and coordination of care.

When the primary nurse is not physically present in the health care facility, patient care is provided by an associate nurse. The associate nurse may be a registered nurse or a licensed practical/vocational nurse.

Functions of a primary nurse include an admission assessment; developing, planning, implementing, and revising the nursing care plan; directing care in his absence; collaborating with physicians and families; making referrals; teaching health concepts; and making discharge plans.

Discussion Questions/Learning Activities

1. Using the hospital in which you will receive the primary portion of your medical and surgical clinical experience, determine who owns the hospital, the kind of service it offers, the number of patient beds, and the average length of stay of most patients.
2. Complete the same information requested in Question 1 for a local nursing home.
3. Make a list of the health care and health-related facilities and services in your local community. (Your local telephone directory is a good place to begin.)
4. In addition to those members of the patient care team discussed in this chapter, how many additional members can you list? Also list their educational preparation and their major function.
5. Obtain an organizational chart for the nursing service department in one of the health care facilities to which you are assigned. How do the job titles of the various members of the nursing department differ from those in Figure 7-2?
6. What nursing care delivery method is used in your clinical affiliation? Is this the same method used in all patient care units in the facility?

References

Aiken LH: Nursing in the 1980s: Crisis, Opportunities, Challenges. Philadelphia, JB Lippincott, 1982.

Ellis JR, Hartley CL: Nursing in Today's World: Challenges, Issues, and Trends. Philadelphia, JB Lippincott, 1988.

Holle ML, Blatchley ME: Introduction to Leadership and Management in Nursing. Boston, Jones and Bartlett, 1987.

Lyon W, Duke BJ: Introduction to Human Services. East Norwalk, CT, Appleton & Lange, 1981.

Potter DO, Rose ME (eds): Practices. Springhouse, PA, Springhouse, 1984.

The Patient: Focus of Nursing Care

8

135

Objectives

When you complete this chapter, you should be able to:

Paraphrase the major rights of patients outlined in "A Patient's Bill of Rights."

Discuss the possible influences of religious convictions on an individual's or a family's health care practices.

Identify some of the differences among patients and how you can meet their nursing care needs.

List some of the precautions that must be taken to maintain a safe environment for patients.

Gwen was aware of the butterflies in her stomach as soon as she opened her eyes that morning. It was her first day on her new job as a licensed practical nurse, and she had a case of the jitters at the thought of putting into practice all she'd been learning this past year. What if she forgot something? "Maybe if I walk to work it will help calm me down," thought Gwen. "Central Memorial Hospital is only 20 minutes away, and it's a lovely day."

Steve Jamison was at his usual spot, watching the neighborhood activity. His wheelchair was drawn up next to his first-floor window so that he could see clearly up and down the street. The disabled man waved to Gwen as she passed. "On your way to school?" he asked.

Gwen smiled. "I graduated last week," she said proudly. "Today's my first day on the job."

"Good luck," Steve called after her.

Gwen heard the shouts of children playing as she approached the playground. She stopped for a minute to watch the lively ball game before she continued on.

A dirty, disheveled woman in a ragged coat and floppy sneakers several sizes too large for her was pawing through a trash can on the corner. "That poor woman could certainly use a bath and some tender loving care," thought Gwen. It seemed she saw more and more such people every day, pushing their shopping carts filled with the castoffs of the city, shouting and mumbling in turn to exorcise their particular demons.

Gwen spotted a small crowd outside the Hill Street Clinic, a small neighborhood health facility. A man was handing out fliers to anyone who would accept them. A young woman attempted to enter the building.

"Abortion is wrong," said the pro-life demonstrator, trying to block the clinic door.

The woman shook her head and quickly slipped past the man into the building. Pro-life demonstrations outside the clinic were a daily occurrence.

Further down the street a volunteer sat at a table collecting signatures of passersby. "Please sign the petition to the Governor asking for additional funds for AIDS research. We need more money to help find a cure."

The man's words sent a chill down Gwen's spine. "AIDS," she thought, "the twentieth-century plague."

"Excuse me," a wistful voice said. "I'm looking for the day care center." It was a young girl with her small child.

Gwen put her hand on the girl's shoulder. "It's across the street," the young nurse said, pointing to a storefront with a simple sign in the window. The girl thanked Gwen and hurried across the street with the child in tow.

In the next block, softly ringing church bells sounded a counterpoint to the traffic noise. Two elderly women reverently entered St. Mary's Church. On the next corner, a bearded young man wearing a skullcap was sweeping the walk in front of the synagogue. He paused to exchange greetings in Hebrew with another man.

As she reached the entrance to Central Memorial Hospital, Gwen thought, "I wonder who my first patient will be?" She recalled each of the people she had seen as she walked to work. She smiled. "It could be anybody."

Pause for a moment and recall the very first time you visited a hospital. It may have been when you were a young child, or later as a teenager. It might have been as recently, such as when you started your practical nursing program. Some people are frequent visitors to the hospital. Others never see the inside of one.

A visit to a hospital or other health care facility can be a very different experience from ordinary daily life for someone who is not accustomed to the routine. The seemingly random movement of physicians, nurses, and other staff members through polished, brightly lighted halls can be puzzling to someone who is uncertain of what to do and where to go. The sights, sounds, and smells are likely to be unfamiliar. The tone of a page, the unexpected appearance of a stretcher, or a sudden flurry of activity can be unsettling.

You are already familiar with your program's facilities or soon will be. Its routine will become more familiar day by day, and you will adapt to it rapidly so that your place in it becomes second nature. You'll ignore most of the background activity and noise, being alert only to your duties and what you must do for the benefit of your patients. Before long, what seemed mysterious and unclear will be as well known to you as the halls of your old high school.

Your patients do not have the benefit of your experience. To them, no matter what their ages, a hospital, clinic, nursing home, physician's office, or almost anyplace where you may be employed may seem strange and possibly frightening. Add the fact that a patient is in a health care facility for a reason, and it becomes clear why you are so important to them. The smile, touch, or kind word of assurance you give them as a caring human being softens the harsh edges of their being there.

The American Hospital Association (AHA) recognized that hospitals are often frightening places and that sometimes both the individual patient and his rights are overlooked by a busy staff. In an effort to remind the health care team to consider patient rights, the AHA published "A Patient's Bill of Rights" in 1973. The full text of this document is found in Appendix H.

Understanding Your Patients

Being a nurse is an enormous responsibility. The best way to fulfill that responsibility is to understand your patients as completely as you can.

Each patient is different from every other. Every one is a distinct, unique human being. An illness or injury may be identical to another, down to the last sign or symptom, but the people who have them are as varied as you can imagine.

However, people do share needs, characteristics, behaviors, customs, and beliefs. When patterns are shared by significant numbers of people, those who share them can be defined as groups. The groups are named by the type of pattern its members share. People can be grouped by age, religion, ethnic background, occupation, or other identifying patterns.

As a nurse, you will always have to be on the alert to treat each of your patients as an individual with individual needs, but you must still be able to care for each one as a member of one or more groups with shared needs.

Cultural and Ethnic Differences

The distinction between cultural and ethnic characteristics and your own personal values and beliefs was made in Chapter 2. "Culture" refers to values and beliefs that are shared by a given group at a given time. "Ethnic" refers to groups sharing customs, language, religion, history, and racial similarities.

Unlike opinions, preferences, and attitudes, which change, cultural and ethnic characteristics are deeply rooted and are difficult or impossible to alter. They are tightly woven into an individual's personality and character. Your patients reflect their cultural and ethnic heritage each time they interact with the world around them. In a situation that is alien to them—a health care setting, for example—their differences may seem magnified, because in stressful situations, most people cling more tightly to what they are familiar with in order to protect themselves against the unknown. Understanding that your patients have differences *and allowing them to have differences without making judgments* are important aspects of being a nurse.

Ethnic grouping is made on the basis of a number of factors—generally race, religion, language, and nationality. You will meet patients who represent a wide variety of each. Some patients will be similar to you, whereas others will be vastly different. Each factor can bear on how the patient relates to the health care setting, particularly where ethnic health care traditions are strong.

There are three major racial divisions—white, black and Asian—each with a number of subgroups. Distinctions among races are physical, such as skin, eyes, hair color and hair texture, and nose and lip shape. These are genetic differences, not cultural or behavioral.

Language is common to everyone, but not everyone shares the same language. Language is a cultural difference among people that can lead to misunderstanding. The problem lies with not understanding the language, not with the fact that languages differ. When a patient speaks a different language or speaks English with an accent, it does not mean his needs are different. It only means that his language differs. When a patient's language difference is enough to seriously limit communication and understanding, find another way to open communication. Loneliness and the fear that accompanies being lonely are difficult enough for a patient to manage. Not being understood adds to a patient's sense of isolation and is unnecessary.

The United States is a "melting pot" of many different nationalities. People from other countries have characteristics that may be very different from your own or those you're familiar with. But differences based on national origin should not be any more of a barrier between you and your patient than different languages are.

People react to circumstances according to how they have learned to react to them in their own culture. Their customs and habits reflect behavior that is correct in their own culture. Their reaction may conflict with what is correct or expected in a different culture. At those times when you and your patient have different points of view because the patient has trouble adapting to the requirements of a health care setting, find someone to act as an "interpreter" to explain the differences.

Religion

Religion is another area of individual preference that must be accommodated in any health care setting. It can be an especially sensitive issue because religious beliefs are among the most fundamental beliefs people have. Persons who are facing immediate, very real questions of health, life, and death will frequently turn to their religion for answers. Circumstances in a hospital, nursing home, or other health care setting can make it difficult for patients to continue their religious practice. No one should stand between the patient and his beliefs. Every opportunity should be available to allow the patient the opportunity to express them. This includes extending an open mind and every courtesy to the patient's priest, minister, rabbi, or other religious representative.

The three major faiths—by population—in the United States are Catholicism, Protestantism, and Judaism. There are many other religions that are not as large in numbers but are just as significant to those who practice them. It is important to remember that to each of your patients, his religion is *the* religion. Remember, too, that many people do not belong to organized religious groups and may not practice or acknowledge any established religion. This does not mean they are antireligion or not religious.

Although you cannot be expected to know all the differences among the many religions and religious denominations, it will be helpful to you to learn the specific needs of your individual patients' religions. A description of some religious practices of some religions follows. In the case of lesser known religions, ask your patient what you can do to make it easier for him to practice his beliefs.

Catholicism

The basic tenet of the Catholic religion is that God, as Jesus Christ, lived and died as a human being so that all of humankind can attain eternal salvation. Various rites known as sacraments (sacred) are performed at appropriate times in the life of Catholics by priests of the church. It is important that a priest or the local Catholic parish be notified as soon as a patient is admitted to the facility, if the patient so desires. This does not imply that the patient is in danger but is a courtesy to the patient. Among the sacraments you may encounter in a health care setting are anointing of the sick, baptism, the Eucharist, and confession and last rites.

One sacrament, baptism, is administered only once in a Catholic's life. Your first obligation to your patient is to call for a priest. Do this regardless of the hour. It is preferable that patients receive sacraments while conscious and unsedated, so the earlier a priest is notified, the better. If a priest is not available, seek a Catholic staff member. As a final resort, you may baptize a patient who has not been baptized and who requests it, or in the case of an unbaptized infant, when asked by a parent.

The form to follow for the sacrament of baptism is to pour water over the patient's forehead or other area of exposed skin at the same time you recite aloud: "I baptize you in the name of the Father, and of the Son, and of the Holy Spirit." Inform the hospital chaplain, the patient's family, or the patient's priest that you administered an emergency baptism and record the fact in nursing notes on the patient's chart.

Eucharist is also called the Holy Eucharist or Communion. A patient preparing to take Communion is required to abstain from food or drink for an hour before the rite, although water and medications are allowed at any

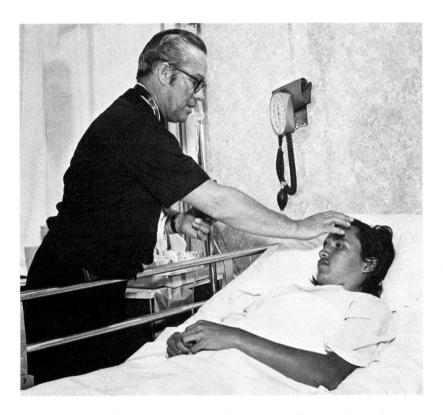

The sacrament for the sick, administered by a Catholic priest, provides comfort.

time. If a patient is unable to attend church or chapel, Communion may be brought to him. Also, if a patient requests Communion preceding surgery, inform your supervisor, the chaplain, or the patient's priest.

Confession is a rite for the forgiveness of sins. The patient's confession is heard by a priest, who then pronounces absolution. It is a very private matter and should be respected as such.

The sacrament of the sick, in which the patient is anointed with holy oil, is frequently misinterpreted as "the last rites" given to someone facing imminent death. This is not the case, and most Catholic families understand this. However, assurances to the patient's family and others that the sacrament is intended for the restoration of physical and spiritual health and is not a preparation for death will help dispel fear and misunderstanding.

Protestantism

A number of separate denominations—over 1200—constitute the faith known as Protestantism. Adherents include Baptists, Episcopalians, Lutherans, Methodists, Presbyterians, members of the United Church of Christ, and Seventh-Day Adventists. A number of their practices differ, although they share many others in common.

Baptists do not practice infant baptism. For them, baptism is a rite to be given only after a believer confesses his faith. They believe that this can be done only by someone who is old enough to understand the significance of baptism. Baptism is by full immersion in water, rather than by sprinkling. Baptists believe that Christ is the head of their church.

Episcopalianism has a number of similarities with Catholicism, including confession, anointing the sick (Holy Unction), Communion, and baptism, although each differs somewhat. Holy Unction, for example, is more often given as a healing sacrament, although it is also administered to those facing death. Episcopalians believe that a dying infant should be baptized, and you may perform a baptism by following the same procedure described for Catholics. The usual administration of these sacraments is by Episcopal priests.

Lutherans practice baptism of children and adults by sprinkling. They also celebrate Communion, at which they believe Christ is present in spirit. Personal faith plays an essential role in their religion, which holds that Christ is both God and man.

Methodists acknowledge the baptismal rites of other religions and practice both infant and adult baptism by sprinkling and by immersion in water. For them, religion is a matter of personal belief, and they use conscience as a guide for living.

Communion (at which Christ is believed to be present in spirit) and baptism (generally by sprinkling) are also practiced by *Presbyterians.* Salvation is believed to be a gift from God.

Members of the *United Church of Christ* practice infant baptism and communion.

Seventh-Day Adventists do not believe in infant baptism. They practice public and private worship, as well as private and group Bible reading. They are generally vegetarians, although some may eat meats that are specified in the Bible. This preference should be respected in the health care setting and notification given to your supervisor or to the dietary department.

Judaism

Judaism, which is the religion and a way of life for Jewish people, is based on the five books of Moses, called the Torah. Culture and religion are deeply intertwined in the Jewish faith. As a result, ritual, tradition, ceremony, religious and social laws, and the observance of holy days (holidays) are often major influences in Jewish daily life.

There are three groups in Judaism: Orthodox, Conservative, and Reform. Although all share the fundamental teachings of Judaism, they vary in how strictly they follow the traditions. Orthodox Jews are the strictest in following Jewish tradition. The Conservative group is less strict, and the Reform group even less rigid.

The rabbi is the spiritual head of a Jewish congregation and is the representative to inform when a patient of the Jewish faith who is admitted to a health care facility requests it.

Because there is a wide difference among Jews in the observance of the customs, rituals, and laws of Judaism, ask your Jewish patients what their preferences are. As always, as with any patient of any religion, belief, or background, when you show a genuine interest and a willingness to personally care for their needs—physical, emotional, and spiritual—they will respond.

A number of Jewish holidays are observed throughout the year. They include Yom Kippur, Rosh Hashanah, Succoth, Hanukkah, and Passover. Each begins at sunset of the day before the holiday and ends at sunset of the next day, or in the case of holidays lasting more than 1 day, at sunset of the last day.

Yom Kippur (Day of Atonement) is Judaism's major holiday. It is celebrated in the fall, 10 days after Rosh Hashanah, the Jewish New Year. Succoth, the Jewish Festival of Thanksgiving, also is celebrated in the fall at about the same time as the American Thanksgiving Day. Hanukkah is an 8-day holiday, also called the Festival of Lights because of the lighting, one by one, of candles on a menorah, a special holiday candleholder. Hanukkah falls in December, generally near Christmas. Passover, also an 8-day holiday, comes in the spring, close to the Christian Easter.

The Jewish Sabbath, a day devoted to prayer, study, and rest, begins at sunset on each Friday and lasts until sunset Saturday. The Sabbath meal is an important occasion.

Circumcision, a religious custom in Judaism, is performed on male infants 8 days after birth by a pediatrician or a rabbi. In some instances the procedure is done by Jewish religious representatives specially trained for the ritual. Jewish boys receive their name at this ceremony. Jewish girls receive theirs at their parents' synagogue (house of worship).

Dietary practices vary among the three Jewish groups. The practices are derived from traditional observances dating from early Jewish history. Kosher—meaning clean or fit to be eaten—restrictions apply to meats, fish, and dairy products and to the utensils they are prepared and served in. The dietary department in health care facilities will observe these restrictions for your patients when they are informed to do so.

Various procedures regarding death are observed in Judaism, though not all by each of the three groups. Generally, all believe that a dying person should not be left alone. Autopsies and embalming are not allowed by Orthodox and Conservative Jews. Funerals are held on the day after the person dies, before sundown, but burial on the Sabbath and some holidays is not permitted.

Other Religions

Members of other Christian denominations you may meet include those belonging to the Eastern Orthodox Church, Jehovah's Witnesses, Friends (Quakers), the Church of Jesus Christ of Latter Day Saints (Mormons), and Christian Scientists. Non-Christian religions include Judaism, Islam (Muslims and Black Muslims), and Buddhism.

Jehovah's Witnesses are prohibited from receiving any blood or blood products.

Mormons, members of the Church of Jesus Christ of Latter Day Saints, do not believe in baptizing infants or in the use of tea, coffee, cola drinks, alcohol, or tobacco.

The religion of *Muslims* (also, *Moslems*) is Islam. Islam holds that Allah is the supreme deity and that Mohammed, the founder of Islam, is the chief prophet. Moslems are forbidden to eat pork in any form or to use alcoholic beverages.

Black Muslims are members of the World Community of Al-Islam, a predominantly black religious group. They have strict dietary, dress, and personal relationship codes.

The *Eastern Orthodox Church* is similar in many respects to the Roman Catholic Church. Find out your patient's preferences before requesting a priest or other church representative for adherents.

In all religions, the patient's religious representative should always be informed that the patient has entered your health care facility, when requested by the patient and when circumstances suggest that spiritual counseling is required. The best way to ensure that this important need is not overlooked is to learn from the patient what his wishes are. It's perfectly appropriate to ask, and it also shows your concern for the whole person beyond his or her immediate physical and medical needs.

Patient Differences

The tendency to categorize people is common. It is sometimes easier to deal with the needs of individuals in a group that shares characteristics or patterns of behavior by assuming that every member of the group has the same needs. In general, this is true. Most children, for example, are frightened by their first experience in a hospital setting. Thus you can assume that any child who comes under your care might be afraid. It is better to make that assumption, and treat the child as though he might be afraid than to neglect the possibility. If it turns out he's not afraid, no harm has been done. If he is, you will be prepared to help him deal with the fear.

Other groups of patients may invite similar assumptions. However, it is important to be careful about making assumptions regarding your patients, because no matter how a person may be categorized, each one is an individual. You will do a better job and feel better about it if you treat each of your patients as a unique human being with special needs. Still, you might consider the following general guidelines when working with certain groups of patients.

The Child

Children may experience a lot of fear in their lives because so much of what they do is new to them. Not all fear is registered as open-eyed trembling. In a hospital or other health care setting, a child may appear to be perfectly normal, sitting quietly or doing just what he's told. Or he may scream and fight any efforts to hold him, especially when facing a procedure that might hurt, such as having blood drawn. In either case, the child may be fearful but may express it in entirely different ways.

Talking to a child to determine whether he is afraid may not work, because a very young child, or one who is very frightened, may not be able to communicate effectively. A nod or a shake of the head from the child will

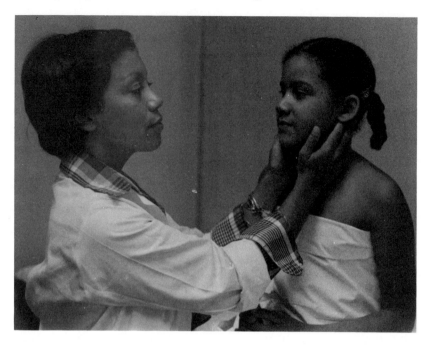

Quiet reassurance from the nurse calms fears.

not provide enough information if you have to make a clinical judgment about what's going on for that child.

To make things easier for you and for your young patients, you must try to make them feel more secure by being warm, open, friendly, and unthreatening. Although you are not a relative or even a family friend, you may be in an excellent position to help a child ward off or calm fears. Holding, touching, and praising a child, and attempting to reduce fear by quiet reassurance, are the kinds of behaviors a child should get from a parent. When a parent is not present, those needs remain. You may be able to meet at least some of them to a certain extent.

When parents or relatives are present, you can be equally important to the child's well-being by providing the human touch that many perceive as missing in a health care setting. A smile, an answered question, reassurance, and a willingness to listen to parents' concerns can help to smooth the way for the child's recovery.

At some time you may find yourself caring for a child who has been abused. Abused children who are hospitalized need more love and attention than any others. They may have an induced fear of adults that could be overwhelming when combined with the normal fear some children have of hospitals and other health care settings. Consult with your instructor or supervisor when an abused child is in your care.

The Elderly Person

Although Americans' understanding of elderly persons has improved greatly, there are still some preconceptions that can make caring for elderly patients difficult. An older person is not a child. Old people are not "senile." They are not hopeless, obstinate, demanding, confused, irrational, or any of a dozen or more other characterizations frequently made about them. It's true that some elderly persons have ailments, that some get sick, and that some react slower than a younger person would. But these things are true for every elderly person—or even for aging people in general. Each one is an individual and must be treated as such.

It is important to understand that as a consequence of a long life, many changes occur in people. Also, the older one gets, the more losses one experiences. A partial loss of hearing or reduced vision certainly affects the older person. Losses may be serious—for example, the loss of a spouse through death. In general, you may assume that any elderly person has suffered some losses. Therefore it is more important than ever for you to treat your older patients in a manner that will reduce further loss. Simple things such as the loss of privacy may not affect a younger patient, but an older patient who loses privacy may be losing one of the few important things he has left.

Independence is a strong characteristic of people in a free society. Institutionalization (being hospitalized or confined to a health care facility such as a nursing home), by its nature, reduces one's independence. To limit elderly patients' independence further by treating them as though they're unable to do anything for themselves is a serious blow. An older patient may need help, and your responsibility is to provide it. But don't make the assumption that just because the patient has gray hair or walks slower than you, he is totally dependent. Learn by observing and by asking your older patients what you can do to help them.

For many reasons, the elderly persons you meet in a hospital setting may show more than average loneliness, depression, confusion, and a sense of being rejected. In many cases these symptoms have causes that can be alleviated. For example, it is not uncommon for elderly persons to neglect their diet. Certain dietary deficiencies can produce depression. Careful assessment may provide clues to the cause of depression.

Elderly persons constitute a highly visible population in health care settings, and of course, they are virtually the entire population in nursing

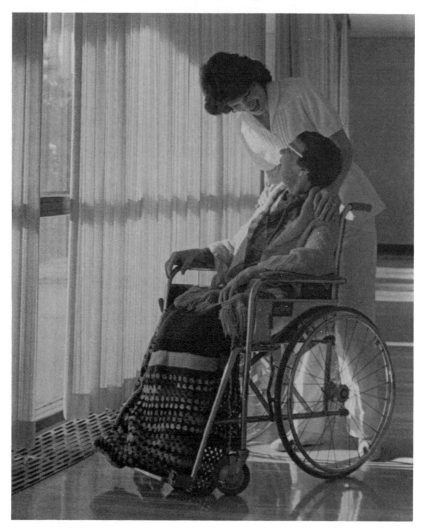

Communication skills are adapted to meet individual patient needs.

homes. The elderly population is growing very rapidly, and the likelihood is that you will encounter more older patients than young ones in your nursing practice. It will be to your benefit to closely study aging and its associated factors. Greater understanding and knowledge will help improve your relationships with older patients, assist you in making clinical decisions in helping older patients, and increase your career opportunities.

The Patient Having an Abortion

An abortion—spontaneous or induced—terminates (ends) a pregnancy before the fetus has developed well enough to live if born.

A spontaneous abortion is a natural termination (ending) of a pregnancy before the twentieth week of gestation. It generally occurs because of problems associated with conception or the maternal environment.

An induced abortion is a medical procedure that intentionally terminates a pregnancy, either at the mother's request or for medical reasons.

Abortions are a combination of a physical event (the abortion itself) and the postabortion period that follows. They are often emotionally charged events in a woman's life and can be very upsetting. A nurse caring for an abortion patient should provide extraordinary understanding along with the routine nursing care required.

There are many facets associated with abortion, including legal, medical, religious, social, emotional, family, and other concerns. You are not expected to be a specialist in these areas, but compassionate understanding in all of them is important.

Regardless of your personal feelings about abortion, it is legal in the United States. Although, as a nurse, you are required to provide nursing care, you may be exempt from assisting with this procedure. There are differences in state abortion laws. You can learn what they are in your state by asking your instructor or the legal representative of your health care facility after you are employed.

The Unmarried Mother

Pregnancies outside of marriage have increased significantly, particularly among adolescents. The phrase "children having children" reflects a real situation. The problems and concerns associated with pregnancy are much greater for young, unwed mothers than for adult women. Not all pregnancies of unmarried girls and women are unwanted, but the majority are.

There are many social implications of unwanted prengancies, whether they are terminated by abortion or brought to term. The mother—especially the young mother—undergoes a considerable amount of emotional stress. She may face social, family, and personal scrutiny and criticism that can be overwhelming.

Regardless of whether an unwed pregnancy is accepted by the mother (and others) or not, it should be assumed there may be underlying emotions that the mother, her family, and others associated with her may be feeling but not expressing. You should treat this situation delicately and be prepared to provide understanding and a willingness to listen at any time. Be certain that your instructor is informed of any behavior changes you see in your patient, and if the situation develops beyond your experience or capacity to manage, be sure that a qualified professional is notified.

The Patient Who Is Homosexual

For many years, homosexuality was so carefully hidden that virtually no one could say with certainty who was homosexual and who was not. With the openness that is now common, male and female homosexuals are less likely to hide their sexual preference, although many still do.

A patient may tell you he or she is homosexual, or you may learn it through other sources. The important thing to keep in mind when you are caring for a homosexual patient is that your obligation is to the patient as a person who requires medical treatment in a health care setting. The homosexuality has nothing at all to do with the nursing care you give.

If you have a patient who tells you that he or she is homosexual, acknowledge it and discuss it freely. Let the patient be the guide to how much discussion is permissible, because privacy is a right of all patients.

The issue of homosexuality has taken on new dimensions as a result of acquired immune deficiency syndrome (AIDS). Many AIDS patients are homosexual. However, it must be underscored that a patient with this disease is not automatically homosexual. Heterosexuals, children, hemophilia patients, and intravenous drug users are also AIDS victims.

There are no medical or legal distinctions to categorize homosexuals, and you owe it to your patient not to make any of your own.

The Patient Who Is Mentally Ill

Everyone has an emotional as well as a physical side. When both are in relative balance, the person is considered well. When either one or both are not balanced, the person is ill. Emotional or mental illness is a disease and must be treated as such. There is no place in a health care setting for terms such as "crazy," "loony," or "nuts," when one is describing a patient or a patient's condition.

There are many health care facilities in the United States devoted exclusively to the care and treatment of mentally ill patients. However, many hospitals have psychiatric units, and any patient may have emotional problems and illness at the same time.

Patients with emotional problems may be admitted for their medical problems or for their psychiatric condition. As a nurse, you will surely encounter emotionally disturbed patients. Your compassion and understanding are powerful tools for their welfare and improvement.

A health care facility may have an effect on people's emotional states.

For example, someone who is facing a life-threatening situation but who is otherwise emotionally stable may become depressed. Or a patient who is anticipating major surgery may become extremely anxious. Someone whose lab test results could affect the rest of his life might withdraw into a shell while waiting. And patients with known psychiatric conditions may get worse—a depression may deepen to thoughts of suicide, for example.

Not all expressions of emotion are clinical, that is, with psychiatrically verifiable pathology (causes). An elderly patient with no relatives, who has no visitors and spends the day wistfully in her room, may say, "I might as well be dead." Such statements do not always represent feelings of suicide, but they should always be noted to your instructor. Often they are cries for attention. You should not be the one to judge whether a patient's expressions of wanting to die are suicidal or are statements of loneliness. In either case, if you respond with warmth, openness, and friendliness, your patient will benefit.

The Patient Who Is Undemanding

Patients in a health care setting who require only minimal nursing care may ask for very little more than what they need. But it is a disservice to any patient to overlook him because he doesn't clamor for attention or mention a need. For example, an elderly patient who is lying on a painful decubitus ulcer may suffer in silence rather than "impose" on you, or a patient who has soiled the bed may be too embarrassed to ask for help.

To avoid these and other situations in which nursing care is needed but may not be reported by the patient, you must take the initiative with all of your patients to bring them into your confidence when you are with them. Let them know that it is okay to tell you what is going on with them, what they need, and what they would like. If you're open and direct with your patients, those who might otherwise go unnoticed will get the full benefit of your care.

The Patient Who Is Hostile

There's another kind of patient in a health care setting who is anything but unnoticed. He or she is the opposite of the shy, undemanding patient and may be disruptive as well. The disruption may be merely vocal, or it may also be physical. The solution is not to avoid the demanding shouts, grumbling complaints, or overt physical acts that are meant to get your attention, but to deal with the patient calmly. Avoid either fueling the situation by collapsing to the demands or fanning it hotter by becoming angry.

Disruptive, complaining behavior is often a cry for attention. If you and your instructor can determine the underlying cause and satisfy the need, the patient will probably calm down. Seriously disruptive behavior should be reported, because it may indicate deeper problems than just a lack of attention.

When behavior becomes truly abusive or hostile, and you, other patients or staff, or the patient himself is threatened with harm, the matter should be reported immediately to your supervisor. If the behavior is violent, as in the case of someone who is mentally disturbed or who is reacting to alcohol or drug abuse, protect yourself and other patients and call for help at once. Don't attempt to restrain a patient who is violent or threatening violence.

The Patient Who Abuses Alcohol or Drugs

The substance-abusing patient may have psychological, medical, and legal problems all at the same time. People do not become addicted to drugs for pleasure or because they're thrilled with how their lives are going. They have underlying needs that are being inappropriately met through chemical interventions that eventually became addictive.

Your duty as a nurse is to provide the care any patient needs, no matter what it was that got him into your care in the first place. Most people have very strong feelings about substance abuse. Yours may be even greater because of what you see in a health care setting. You must not let those feelings come between you and your patient, as difficult as this may be. Substance abuse is a disease and must be treated as such. Sometimes the consequences of a substance abuser's acts may cause outrage—for example, a drunk driver may run over and kill a child. It will take an exceptionally strong commitment on your part, but you cannot turn your back on the abuser, any more than you could on the child if he survived.

Any person with a diagnosis of substance abuse needs more care than you alone can give. If your patient is not already under special care for substance abuse, help to see that he gets such care by informing your instructor of the need and by providing information to the patient or the patient's family about where such care can be obtained.

The Patient Who Is Dying

A goal of health care is to improve life, but dying and death are facts that cannot be overlooked by health care personnel. The number of dying patients that you will care for will depend on the type of work you do after you enter practice. In some fields, death is very remote, whereas in others it is a regular occurrence. You may never get used to working with dying patients, but there are ways to make the situation more comfortable for your patients, their families, and yourself.

When you are caring for someone who is dying, the most important thing you can do for him is to be secure with your own feelings. Helping your patients will depend on your ability to be objective about their situation in the midst of an emotionally wrenching series of predictable events while maintaining and expressing honest concern for their welfare.

Being objective does not mean being indifferent, but you need to remain apart from the turmoil of death so that you can see clearly what is needed and what you must do. This places a very large demand on you.

Death in a health care setting comes in two general ways: expected, as in the case of terminally ill patients, and unexpected, as in the case of accident victims, heart attack victims, and others who, except for the immediate cause, would not have died. The latter group includes patients who die suddenly during an otherwise positive recovery.

Little can be done to prepare for unexpected deaths except to know they will happen, and when they do, to get past your own shock and disbelief so that you can continue to function for your other patients and also provide solace for the family and friends of the deceased.

A patient who is known to be dying—as in the case of someone with a long-term illness—will pass through a series of stages that, if completed, will prepare them for death. Dr. Elizabeth Kübler-Ross distinguished five stages of dying in her book *On Death and Dying*: denial, anger, bargaining, depression, and acceptance.

The first stage, denial, may last a short or a long time. It expresses the patient's unwillingness to accept a serious illness and its likely consequences.

When the reality of what is happening can no longer be denied, the patient will become angry. He may show this anger by being demanding, difficult, critical, and unpleasant. This second stage may be difficult for you to deal with because one reaction to someone who is being objectionable is to respond in the same way. You must not. It is here that your objectivity will get you through. The patient's behavior toward you is not personal, though it may sound as though it is. Realize that the patient must express this anger in order to progress toward full acceptance of events he cannot control.

As the patient understands more fully that death is inevitable, he may bargain for time. He may make promises. Sometimes the promises are made to society, to God, to a church, or to someone on the hospital staff. They can take any form, but the offer is usually to exchange something—a donation to a cause, a promise to be good—for more life.

When it is even more clear that nothing can be done to change what is happening, the patient may become depressed. He may cry. He may be silent. At first he may mourn past events in his life—those things he thinks he should have done differently, or losses he's already experienced. This kind of depression is similar to that which everyone has from time to time.

As time passes, the nature of the patient's depression changes as he begins to mourn his own death. It is a grief that cannot be shared, because the dying patient is grieving over the impending loss of *everyone*, and only someone who is dying can know what that must be like. However, the patient must be allowed to express this grief. You can encourage this expression by making it okay for him to cry or to talk about his grief if he chooses.

If the preceding stages are allowed to be completed by the patient, and when his denial, anger, bargaining, and grief are finished, he may reach the stage of acceptance. Acceptance of death does not mean willingness to die, but it does mean that the patient is in some way ready.

Dr. Kübler-Ross says that all patients know when they are terminally ill, even if they have not been told. It is not your responsibility to inform a patient that he is dying, but your ability to help him through the dying process will be improved if you know what he knows about his condition. Ask your instructor or supervisor whether your patient has been told he is dying. If he has, you can deal with the situation openly.

In the course of a terminally ill patient's care, you will also get to know family, friends, and other regular visitors. They may rely on you for information, for trust, and as someone to whom they can express their feelings. Your best preparation is to have a thorough understanding of your own feelings and the knowledge that you can interact with compassion while maintaining the required objectivity that allows you to function efficiently.

Visitors: Family and Friends

Most patients in a health care facility welcome visitors, but some have no visitors. For those without visitors, you and your co-workers become substitutes for the family, relatives, and friends who might otherwise stop in to see them.

Most patients will have visitors. Their presence and how they interact with the patient and the facility staff can have a major effect on the patient's recovery. The effect can be positive or negative. As an objective but concerned party to the patient's welfare, you can influence what that effect will be by creating a positive relationship with your patient's visitors. By being open, friendly, courteous, kind, and otherwise responsive to the visitor's concerns, you will instill a feeling of trust.

Being friendly does not mean that you give up your authority when the patient's best interest is in question. You must remain firm and persuasive when visiting hours are over, when a distraught visitor would do more harm than good, if a scheduled procedure requires the visitors to leave, and in other situations where your duties supersede visitors' wishes. Yet you must demonstrate your authority in a pleasant way, even when the visitor resorts to unpleasantness.

Always respect your patient's privacy. If your duties can wait while visitors are present, avoid disturbing them. On the other hand, if your nursing care is required, you must direct the visitors to leave if the situation warrants—for example, if the patient has to be exposed.

Consult with your instructor regarding policies on visiting hours, when a patient can receive visitors, how many visitors are allowed, and other restrictions. When problems arise that you are unable to correct, ask your instructor for assistance.

Nurse-Patient Interaction

Of all the considerations regarding you and your patient, the most important is the personal relationship between you. The guidelines and regulations governing your duties will be set by your program. Your role as student nurse is acknowledged. How you fulfill it as you give nursing care to your patients is an individual matter.

Two principal influences that will affect the skill with which you deliver nursing care are your education and your self-confidence. As you study, you are building a base of information and experience that you will use when you enter practice. Your education will be the basis for the care you will give. However, without confidence in your ability and a good understanding of yourself, you may be reluctant to use what you have learned.

Your confidence in yourself and your skills will be what cements your relationships with your patients. Knowing who you are and what you can do will help you to be objectively aware of your patient, his needs, and his concerns. At the same time, you will be able to draw on your own feelings to relate to your patient as another human being who cares and understands. The nurse who is shy, insecure, self-serving, or more concerned with meeting her own needs than her patients' needs will not be able to give the care they need and expect. Your first obligation—after your commitment to getting the best education you can—is to develop a self-awareness that will allow you to interact with your patients as a skilled, informed nurse and a sensitive, caring human being.

Sympathy and empathy are distinctly different feelings. Your effectiveness in relating to your patients requires that you have a clear understanding of the difference. Without it, you will not be able to grasp the significance of your patient's condition and its meaning to him. Empathy allows you to remain outside the condition, not to be drawn into it. You have to know what impact the illness will have on the patient's life so that you can help him to live with it. You must also understand the medical implications of your patient's illness so that your observations and reporting of his condition and its changes will be meaningful, and so that when you carry out treatment orders, you will do so appropriately.

Patient Safety

An irony of hospitalization is that a patient may be in danger by being there. Health care facilities are complex. They are filled with people in constant activity. They are equipped with machines and electronic devices. A wide variety of combustible materials, including flammable liquids and gases, are everywhere. The potential for an accident or a fire is never far away, and patients—dependent on you and others for their physical safety—are in the middle of it all.

Learn the fire and safety regulations of the facility you serve. Know the locations of all exits. Personally check where fire extinguishers are kept so that you know where to get one if needed. Mention any safety problem, no matter how small, to your team leader. A loose wire, a lamp that sputters, a peculiar smell, a loose bed rail, a slippery spot on the floor, or a machine that feels hot but shouldn't is not too insignificant to report.

If you do smell smoke or see flames, immediately follow the procedure set by your facility's regulations. Don't attempt to put out a fire without first informing the appropriate person or giving the required alarm. Don't panic. Your patients will need you in the event an evacuation is necessary.

Other aspects of patient safety may be less apparent; however, they are just as important. Be sure the patient has an identification bracelet on his wrist. Check the name on the bracelet to be sure you are administering medications or treatments to the right patient. Be sure that medical supplies are removed after treatments or procedures are completed. A needle or other potentially dangerous piece of equipment left in the patient's bed or in his room can cause serious injury.

Clean up spills when they occur. Not only might a spill cause a patient to slip and fall, but nurses and others may also fall. Close doors and drawers when you are finished. Many an injury has been caused by tripping over open cabinet doors or bumping into the corner of an open door.

Know whether it is required that bed rails be up for a particular patient. If they are to be up, be sure you leave them up when you leave the patient's room. This is especially true for children in cribs. If the height of the bed is adjustable, be sure it is in the low position before you leave the patient.

If restraints are ordered to prevent a patient from injuring himself, be sure they are snug but not too tight. Check the patient frequently to be sure restraints have not constricted circulation.

There are many opportunities in the hospital for accidents to occur. Use common sense, look around you, and accept personal responsibility for correcting situations that could lead to accidents and injury. Don't wait to be told to take action. If a situation is beyond your ability to correct—a frayed electrical cord, for example—be sure you report it to your instructor or other appropriate person. Then be persistent so that the situation that needs correcting is not forgotten.

Discussion Questions/Learning Activities

1. Think about the following situation: A 35-year-old man is admitted to the emergency room of a short-term ("acute") care hospital after an automobile accident. He was alone in the car, his family and home are in a city 100 miles away, and he has never been in the hospital before. His most serious injury appears to be a broken leg; however, the doctors are considering the possibility of internal injuries. What do you think some of his thoughts and feelings might be while he is waiting for their diagnosis? How might you as a student nurse help this patient during this crisis?

2. Cultural and ethnic differences exist in almost every group. What are some of the cultural and ethnic differences of students in your class?

3. How many different religious organizations are there in your community? You might begin by using the telephone directory.

4. Several special groups of patients were discussed in this chapter. Think of a group or category of patient not discussed and outline some of the more significant characteristics of that group.

5. What are some of the things you could do to make a hospital stay more pleasant for a patient who has no visitors?

6. Suppose a patient is attempting to become friendly with you or even asks you to go out on a date. What are some of the techniques you might use to handle this situation?

7. You see an employee who is waiting for the elevator spill some water on the floor. The employee realizes what she did, but the elevator doors open and she gets on the elevator. What will you do?

References

American Nurses' Association. Contemporary Minority Leaders in Nursing: Afro-American, Hispanic, Native American Perspectives. New York, The Association, 1983.

Henderson G, Primeaux M: Transcultural Health Care. Menlo Park, CA, Addison-Wesley, 1981.

Joos IR, Nelson R, Lyness RN: Man, Health, and Nursing: Basic Concepts and Theories. East Norwalk, CT, Appleton & Lange, 1985.

Kübler-Ross E: Questions and Answers on Death and Dying. New York, Macmillan, 1974.

Kübler-Ross E: Living With Dying. New York, Macmillan, 1981.

Lindberg JB: Introduction to Person-Centered Nursing. Philadelphia, JB Lippincott, 1983.

Milliken ME: Understanding Human Behavior. Albany, NY, Delmar, 1981.

Murray RB, Zentner JP: Nursing Concepts for Health Promotion. East Norwalk, CT, Appleton & Lange, 1985.

Spector RE: Cultural Diversity in Health and Illness. East Norwalk, CT, Appleton & Lange, 1985.

Ethical Issues in Health Care

9

Objectives

When you complete this chapter, you should be able to:

Define the word "ethical."

Describe the three areas in which ethical decisions are made.

Explain why a study of ethics and ethical behavior is important in nursing.

State the purposes of a code of ethics.

Paraphrase the NFLPN and the NAPNES statements regarding ethical behavior of practical/vocational nurses.

Explain personal responsibility and accountability as it relates to ethical behavior.

Outline the guidelines for making decisions related to ethical concerns.

Debate the pros and cons of a contemporary biomedical ethical issue.

Jim and Jeannie started practical nursing school 2 months ago. They were already good friends, and they often studied together. Jim was doing very well. His lowest grade was a 92. Jeannie was a different story. Her grades were generally poor. In fact, if she did not pass the upcoming exams, she would be terminated from the program.

Jim was concerned for his friend. "The exam is next week," he said. "I'll help you study this weekend, if you like."

"Oh, that's very nice of you, Jim," Jeannie said as they chatted over coffee after their last class on Friday. "I just don't think I'll have time. I have some shopping to do tomorrow. And I've got a date tomorrow night." She thought for a moment. "But Sunday would be fine. Can you call me then to set up a time?"

"I sure will," Jim said. "One day of study is better than none. Especially for you, Jeannie. It could mean your whole nursing career."

Jeannie nodded. "I know," she said. She was very serious.

On Sunday morning, Jim called Jeannie. "What time do you want to meet me?" he asked.

There was silence for a moment. Then Jeannie spoke. "For what?" she said.

"We were going to study for the exam today," Jim said.

"Oh, I can't," Jeannie said. "I didn't get in until early this morning. I'm so tired I can't even think of studying."

"Do you want me to come by later this afternoon?" Jim asked, unwilling to let his friend miss her last opportunity to prepare for the exam.

"Sure," Jeannie said. "That's a good idea."

When Jim went to Jeannie's that afternoon, there was a note on the door. It said: "Jim. I forgot I had to go to my mother's for dinner. See you in class tomorrow. J."

The next day, Jim met Jeannie in the hall. "I left a set of my notes under your door," he said. "Did you get a chance to read them?"

Jeannie smiled. "That was so sweet, Jim. But, I just couldn't find the time. It was late and—to be perfectly honest, I'm not really worried about this exam."

"Well, I am," Jim said. "And I'm only trying to keep my average up. Not keep from getting terminated from the program."

Jeannie squeezed his hand. "You worry too much," she said.

Later, when the class was assembled for the exam, Jim nodded to Jeannie. "Good luck," he said.

"Thanks," she whispered back.

The instructor distributed the exam papers. Jim glanced through it to familiarize himself with its content and to estimate how much time he would need to complete it. Other students did the same, although some started writing their answers immediately.

About halfway through the exam, Jim glanced across the aisle at Jeannie. He was astonished by what he saw. In her hand was a 3 by 5-inch index card. She looked at it and then slipped it out of sight before answering a test question. She did this a number of times during the exam. She was still writing when Jim turned in his paper and left the room.

Jeannie joined him a few minutes later. "That wasn't so hard after all, was it?" she said.

"You didn't think so?" Jim asked in surprise. "Maybe it wasn't the hardest exam we've had, but it sure wasn't the easiest. I know I couldn't have winged it."

Jeannie said nothing.

"Did you get a chance to go over the notes I left?" Jim asked.

Jeannie's hand shot up. "Oh, there's Diana," she said, waving her arm. "I have to talk to her about something. Diana! Wait up!" She turned to Jim. "See you tomorrow."

The hall emptied as the last of the students left the exam room. Soon it was very quiet. Jim was deeply concerned. A flurry of questions raced through his mind. "Did Jeannie cheat on the exam? What should I do? Should I tell her what I saw? Should I ask her if she used notes? Should I report her? Is it my business to snitch on someone if I *think* she cheated? Is it my business to report someone if I *know* they cheated? What if we were on duty and I saw Jeannie do something dishonest that would harm a patient, like writing on a chart that she did something but really didn't? Would I be responsible?" Jim shook his head sharply. "I'll have to make Jeannie talk to me about this," he said to himself.

Jim's conscience was guided by what he and his class had already covered and discussed at great length: the ethical issues that are the concern of everyone who accepts the responsibility of caring for others.

For many years now you have been developing personal standards of conduct and making moral judgments based on your personal beliefs and values. Before you entered nursing school, your personal standards of conduct, your beliefs, your values, and your prejudices probably had little influence on others. Perhaps those who did not agree with your opinions were not your friends; those who did not approve of the way you conducted yourself did not associate with you.

But now that you have decided to become a nurse, you must examine yourself, your heart and your soul, very closely. By becoming a nurse, you agree to provide certain services to human beings. And human beings have certain rights that are absolute. That means that these rights apply equally to every human being. Human rights are absolute privileges that people have and that they have a right to expect because they are human. There are many human rights. Some are specific to individuals; some are specific to groups.

People are not more or no less human because of their income, their occupation, their sex, their race, or any of an infinite number of factors that make people different. Although people are different in what they think, how they behave, the language they speak, and the clothes they wear, certain characteristics are common to all. All humans bleed when they are cut, and all need air, food, and water. All are born, and all die. All have hearts and lungs and livers. In other words, there are certain attributes that are fundamental to all humans.

The fundamental characteristics common to all humans raise certain philosophical questions that have been debated for centuries. What rights does a human being have just because he is human, and what responsibilities are associated with these rights? Ethical questions are directly related to these philosophical questions. The word "ethical" comes from the Greek *ēthikos* and means knowledge of right and wrong related to human conduct. Decisions based on this knowledge of right and wrong may be related to the individual, the society, or the situation.

An individual makes many decisions on the basis of what he or she personally believes is right or wrong. These beliefs begin developing early in life and generally evolve from what a child is taught by his parents, his friends, his culture, his religion, his school, and society in general. This is a personal value system. A healthy individual changes his value system over his lifetime. What he believes about his relationships with, and his responsibilities to, other people changes as he learns and lives in society.

Decisions regarding what is right and what is wrong are also made by society. These decisions may be carried out through changes in customs and behaviors, or they may be written as laws. There are many examples of how society continually redefines right and wrong. Abolition of slavery, the right to vote, and women's rights are just a few examples of how our society has redefined human rights over time. Laws that govern the conduct of societies are written statements that define right and wrong; they will be discussed in Chapter 10. Decisions about what is right and what is wrong can also be situational. That is, what is right in one situation may be wrong in another.

This is by no means an exhaustive discussion of ethics or ethical behavior. You should realize that human beings have fundamental rights and that society gives nurses a responsibility for protecting those rights. Many decisions you make related to your nursing responsibilities to society will involve ethical behavior.

Nursing and Ethics

A study of ethical behavior and nursing is one of the most important aspects of your nursing education. Society has, through nurse licensing laws, given nurses "permission" to nurse other human beings. People who become nurses promise or agree to help all those human beings who need their services. Nurses, by virtue of their education, have the ability and the responsibility to help patients. The public trusts nurses to have the knowledge necessary to be a nurse as well as the moral commitment to fulfill the obligation of nursing.

One of the most important things you should remember is that anyone can learn the knowledge and perform the skills assigned to nursing. But not everyone who has this knowledge and these skills can be called a nurse. A nurse is someone who has internalized the concept of what it means to be a human being and accepts personal responsibility for relationships with other human beings. A nurse makes a moral commitment to provide the same quality and level of nursing service to all human beings.

Your interpretation of what it means to be human, your belief in what rights humans have, and your ideas of what is right and what is wrong are what make you the person you are. And you cannot separate the person you are from the nurse you hope to become. A strong belief in the right of people to be treated and respected as human beings must be the foundation of your relationships and interactions with your patients, with your fellow nurses, and with members of the health care team.

To help you develop ethical behavior so essential to nursing. NFPLN and NAPNES have each developed a code of ethics for practical/vocational nurses. A code of ethics is a list of rules of good conduct for members of a particular group. Although laws establish the minimum behaviors of a group, ethical statements attempt to describe the ideals of that group.

The legal/ethical status section of the Nursing Practice Standards for the Licensed Practical/Vocational Nurse, published by the National Federation of Licensed Practical Nurses (Appendix D), indicates that practical/vocational nurses "shall recognize and have a commitment to meet the ethical and moral obligations of the practice of nursing." The National Association for Practical Nurse Education and Service has also issued a statement regarding ethical behavior and the practical/vocational nurse. The full NAPNES statement appears in Appendix I. Both of these statements identify those standards of behavior that reflect the high ideals of the practical/vocational nurse.

You will be provided with many opportunities during your educational program to acquire the knowledge, skills, and ethical behaviors expected of practical/vocational nurses. Your faculty will assist you in reaching your goal of becoming a nurse. It is through their instruction and guidance that you will learn not only how to bathe a patient but how to accept personal responsibility for what you do. You will learn to recognize that with responsibility comes accountability.

A desire to help others and a moral commitment to be responsible and accountable for your actions is the ethical foundation of your career as a licensed practical/vocational nurse.

Personal Accountability

Being responsible means to accept being the cause of an action. For example, saying "I broke the window" indicates the acceptance of personal responsibility. Being accountable means to accept the consequences of the action—for example, "I will pay for the broken window."

Being held accountable for what you do and how you do it can be the most rewarding part of your career in nursing. You can be proud of how you perform your nursing skills, you can feel great personal satisfaction about the knowledge you gain as you accumulate experiences in nursing, and you can accept the admiration of your peers because of your high moral standards. Your patients will feel your concern for them as individual human beings, and they will remember the kind, caring nurse who helped them through a difficult time in their life.

Unethical Behavior

Unfortunately, not all nurses adhere to their code of ethics. You may see situations in which there is blatant disregard for basic human rights. You may hear patients referred to as the gallbladder in Room 212 or the appendectomy in Room 324. You may see members of the health care team ignoring a patient's questions or generally treating them without respect. You may find yourself working with people who chart procedures that were not done, don't wash their hands properly, ignore isolation procedures, and so forth. Such situations are difficult for you as a person and also for you as a nurse. These ethical dilemmas are not associated with major issues such as organ transplants; they are issues associated with the day-to-day contacts in which some people forget their basic responsibility to society—the very group that gave them the right to practice nursing.

What you choose to do in this situation is a difficult decision. If the majority of the people you work with frequently ignore the human rights of patients, your best decision may be to resign from that position. If the problem is limited to just a few people or one person, your team leader or head nurse may also be concerned. Together, with tact and courage, you may be able to help that nurse perform his or her responsibilities at a level that reflects positively not only on the nurse but on all of nursing.

Guidelines for Making Decisions Related to Ethical Concerns

Ethical concerns of contemporary nurses are varied. They may be related to the more dramatic biomedical ethical issues that will be discussed later in this chapter, but they also include the day-to-day practice of nursing. One of the major concerns is the chemically impaired nurse. Another concern is expressed by nurses who are working in situations where the shortage of nursing staff compromises the quality of patient care. Other concerns are related to poor performance by peers, medication and patient care errors, theft of supplies and equipment, confidentiality of patient information, and a person's right to health care regardless of ability to pay. These are just a few issues. You will no doubt develop other concerns as you become more and more involved in nursing. Each of these issues could be discussed at length, but it is more appropriate to offer general guidelines for handling ethical dilemmas.

Before guidelines are offered for dealing with ethical dilemmas, it is important for the nurse to have a good understanding of the code of ethics, the nurse practice act of the state in which the nurse is working, and the policies and procedures of the institution in which the nurse is employed.

Although these foundations, which were previously reviewed in some detail, are clearly the basis for an effective and rational approach to the question of what is right and what is wrong, they do not provide direct answers to all the ethical questions you may ask.

This first guideline in thinking about a specific situation is to collect the facts. Did you directly observe the situation, or did you get the information from someone else? Did the situation happen once, or does it happen frequently? Was someone's life in danger? Was the quality of patient care compromised? Is the question one of what is right and what is wrong in relation to human beings, or is it a question of what you would personally prefer? These are questions you must answer clearly and factually for yourself.

The second guideline is to ask yourself what would happen if everyone acted or behaved in the manner in question. Your answer to this question may make the right course of action very clear to you.

If your ethical dilemma is not resolved, a third guideline may provide direction. In this step, you discuss your concerns with an authority. The

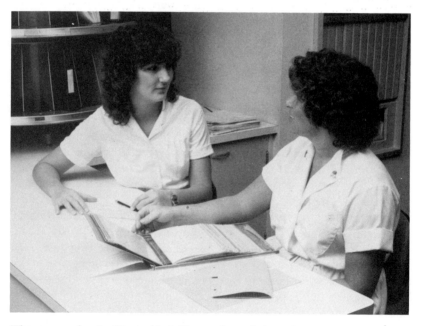

When you are faced with an ethical dilemma, it may help to discuss your concerns with someone with extensive experience and knowledge.

"authority" is someone with extensive experience and knowledge who can help you separate the facts from the emotional components of ethical dilemmas. The discussion process may provide you with new insights, an appreciation of differing points of view, and perhaps even a better understanding of your own values.

After collecting the facts, asking yourself what would happen if everyone behaved in a certain manner, and consulting an authority, you have to choose a course of action. In most cases, your first course of action is to discuss your concerns with your immediate supervisor. This person is often in a position to deal effectively and positively with ethical problems. If, after a reasonable time, you believe that your immediate supervisor has not taken the necessary action to protect the human rights of your patients, you may decide to report your concerns further. Almost all oganizations have lines of authority that you should follow in pursuing your concerns.

Because ethical behavior is difficult to define, particularly when specific situations may justify certain behaviors, a more effective way to present your concerns may be through established institutional committees. The policy and procedures committee, the quality assurance committee, the peer review committee, the patient relations committee, and similar committees may share your concerns. Volunteering to serve on one of these committees or telling your concerns to a member of that committee may be the most effective approach to dealing with your ethical concerns.

When you make a decision to pursue an ethical concern, you must be prepared to accept the consequences of your action. It is possible that other people will not see the situation the same way you see it. You may be labeled a "do-gooder," a "perfectionist," or a "spoiler." Or you may earn the respect of other people. Be sure of your facts and avoid making personal judgments about other people's behavior. Your motivation in pursuing ethical concerns is the protection of the human rights of your patients.

Contemporary Biomedical Ethical Issues

Inherent in being human is the right to make choices. Not that many years ago, choices related to health care were limited. But advances in science and technology in the past 25 years have created many more choices. Organ transplants, advanced life support systems, and alternative methods of conception and contraception are examples of some of the health care options people have today. These options have created ethical dilemmas that you may encounter in your nursing career. And there is no doubt that the future will present us with biomedical ethical issues even more complex that those which are discussed on the following pages.

Birth Control

"Birth control" is the general term used to describe methods of controlling conception. The moral issue over birth control is whether or not individuals have the right to control conception, and if so, what limitations, if any, should be imposed on them.

Limitations include questions regarding which methods are best, what age is appropriate, if methods should be available to married and unmarried people, whether parental consent for minors is needed, and if methods and information should be available through schools or public-supported clinics. Methods of birth control include *contraception, sterilization,* and *elective abortion.*

Contraception prevents fertilization by blocking the union of sperm and egg by means of various devices, spermatocides, or oral contraceptives on a regular basis. When contraception ends, fertilization is again possible.

Sterilization is a surgical procedure that can be performed on men (vasectomy) or women (tubal ligation) to prevent reproduction. It is virtually permanent because neither procedure can be reversed with certainty.

Abortion is the termination of pregnancy. Spontaneous abortion results from abnormalities in the fetus or in the maternal environment and occurs naturally. Elective abortion is intentional, performed at the mother's request and for personal or medical reasons.

Although abortion is legal, it raises numerous ethical issues. There is major controversy regarding the right of women to have control of their own bodies, whether and when a fetus is a human being, and whether a fetus has rights. The U.S. Supreme Court decided the legality of abortion in 1973, but the ethical and moral issues continue. Your personal views will determine whether and to what extent you can comfortably assist in matters relating to abortion.

Alternative Fertilization

For women who cannot conceive, medical techniques now give them the ability to bear children. In addition, men whose fertility was marginal can now father children, and couples can have children through the services of others (*surrogates,* meaning substitutes). These techniques involve artificial insemination, *in vitro,* or "test tube," conception, and surrogate motherhood. All raise legal and ethical questions that remain unanswered.

Artificial insemination is the medical implantation of donor sperm into a woman's uterus to fertilize her own egg and thereby conceive a child. The sperm can be that of the husband or another donor.

Test tube conception is a procedure in which sperm and egg are mixed outside the body in a laboratory dish and the fertilized egg is then implanted into a woman's uterus. The egg and sperm can be from husband and wife, or from donors.

When a fertilized egg is implanted into the uterus of a woman who is not the wife but who will carry the conceived child to term, or when a woman agrees to undergo artificial insemination for another couple, the woman is called a surrogate (substitute) mother.

Some of the legal and ethical questions raised by these methods include the legitimacy of the child, maternal and paternal rights, and adultery. None of them have been fully settled. Your own views will be the basis for your decisions to participate in health care situations in which these issues are raised.

Genetic Screening

Procedures to study genes and to probe the uterus to learn the status of a developing embryo or fetus in order to give physicians, researchers, and parents options and choices that never existed before are methods of genetic screening.

Amniocentesis is a procedure in which a long needle is used to draw amniotic fluid from the sac surrounding the developing child. The fluid can be studied in the laboratory for indications of Down's syndrome, hemophilia, Tay-Sachs disease, Duchenne's muscular dystrophy, sickle cell disease, and other diseases. It can also be used to determine the sex of the unborn infant.

When diseases or genetic abnormalities become known, the parents can be informed and counseled, after which they can decide what to do.

Organ Transplants

The marvel of organ transplantation has become commonplace. Heart, lung, heart and lung, liver, and kidney transplants are done regularly. Recipients of donated organs are given new chances for an improved life and sometimes even for life itself. Living donors, such as those who give one of their kidneys, have the satisfaction that their act has improved someone else's chances for a normal life. The next of kin of deceased donors can take solace from the knowledge that some good has come from their personal tragedy.

In most organ transplants, donor organs come from deceased persons. Some donors make arrangements for organ donation before death through an act of consent in their will, on a special donor card, or by authorization on their driver's license. Other donations are made with the permission of next of kin after the donor's death.

For donated organs to maintain their function after transplantation, they must be removed from the donor as soon after death as possible.

Death

Determining when death occurs has been complicated by lifesaving devices and procedures. Respirators, heart and lung machines, and other assistive devices are able to keep alive patients who a few years ago would have died.

When death is in question, it is now defined on the basis of an electroencephalogram (EEG) when it indicates the absence of brain wave activity. Death is legally defined as the irreversible cessation of brain function for a given period.

Although criteria have been established so that a person can be declared legally dead, it is now possible to continue a deceased patient's biological functions. Therefore the question of whether the patient is alive or dead is still at issue, especially in situations where the removal of the life support system is requested by a next of kin.

Euthanasia

Sometimes called "mercy killing," euthanasia is the deliberate causing of someone's death by active or passive means. Active euthanasia is to cause someone's death by intentionally administering an agent that would bring about death. Passive euthanasia is to cause someone's death by withholding efforts to sustain life.

For example, in a health care setting, an act of active euthanasia could be the administration of a lethal dose of medication, whereas an act of passive euthanasia could be the withholding of a medication that the patient needs to stay alive. Active euthanasia is an unquestionably illegal act (murder) punishable by law. Passive euthanasia is not as well defined, but it is no less controversial.

Living Wills

In some instances, patients anticipate their death and make an allowance to let it happen naturally by signing a living will. A living will is a document that testifies that the patient does not want heroic lifesaving measures instituted to keep him alive when death would otherwise be likely. Living wills are not universally recognized as legal documents, but they do express the wishes, at the time of signing, of those who sign them.

Summary

In summary, learning to be a nurse requires more than passing written examinations and performing procedures correctly. It requires you to develop an ethical and moral commitment to provide the best nursing services you are capable of providing to every human being in your care. This commitment lives within you and cannot be turned on as you begin your nursing duties nor turned off when you leave your patients at the end of your workday. This commitment pervades your life and influences all your decisions. And the longer you are employed as a nurse, the stronger this commitment will become. Nurses who make this personal commitment to their fellow human beings are rewarded by great personal satisfaction; patients who receive nursing services from these nurses are rewarded by compassionate, personal, and competent care.

Discussion Questions/Learning Activities

1. Construct a list of what you believe to be basic human rights. Compare your list with that of one or two of your classmates. Do you agree or do you differ on what constitutes basic human rights? Can you develop a list of basic human rights on which you both agree?

2. Think about your recent experiences in school or in your clinical facility and try to identify an ethical issue. How did you handle this issue, and what do you think you might do if the situation happens again? Indicate why you believe your concern is an ethical one and not a matter of personal values. If you cannot think of your own situation, you may use one of these: cheating on tests; discussing confidential patient information in an elevator; a man's refusing to allow his sick wife to go to a doctor or hospital.

3. Compare and contrast the NAPNES and NFLPN code of ethics. How are they similar? How are they different?

4. Talk with your classmates to determine their position on some of the ethical issues presented in this chapter. Listen to their points of view and compare them with your own. After this discussion, write a brief summary of why you think it is often difficult to find answers to ethical issues.

References

Curtin L, Flaherty MJ: Nursing Ethics: Theories and Pragmatics. East Norwalk, CT, Appleton & Lange, 1981.

Davis A, Aroskar M: Ethical Dilemmas in Nursing Practice. East Norwalk, CT, Appleton & Lange, 1983.

Donnelly GF: The Nursing System: Issues, Ethics and Politics. New York, John Wiley & Sons, 1980.

Potter DO, Rose ME (eds): Practices. Springhouse, PA, Springhouse, 1984.

Purtilo RB, Cassel K: Ethical Dimensions in the Health Professions. Philadelphia, WB Saunders, 1981.

Steele SM, Harmon VM: Values Clarification in Nursing. East Norwalk, CT, Appleton & Lange, 1983.

10 Legally Responsible Nursing Practice

Objectives

When you complete this chapter, you should be able to:

Discuss the purpose of Good Samaritan Laws.

List the two sources of laws and give examples of each.

Discuss the relationship between the nurse practice acts and the state boards of nursing.

Explain the association among responsibility, accountability, and legal liability.

Define the term *respondeat superior.*

Define the term "breach of contract."

Define the term "tort" and give two examples of torts.

Illustrate the difference between a tort and a crime.

Differentiate negligence and gross negligence.

Discuss how nurses can assist in preventing malpractice claims.

Explain the purpose of malpractice insurance.

Give examples of crimes that may involve nurses.

Larry's phone rang a third time. He groped for the receiver. "Hello?" he said drowsily.

"Larry?" a small voice asked. "Please help me. I'm sick."

"Mrs. Thompson, is that you? I'll be right down," Larry said. He raced downstairs to his landlady's apartment.

Mrs. Thompson was lying on the floor next to her bed. Her eyes were closed. Larry dropped to his knees and put his fingertips on the pulse point on the side of her neck. "Mrs. Thompson? Can you hear me?"

The sick woman's eyes opened weakly. Her mouth moved, but there was no sound before she lapsed into unconsciousness again. Larry quickly dialed the phone.

A shadow appeared in the open doorway as he waited for the call to go through. "What happened?" It was Milo Davis, the other tenant in Mrs. Thompson's building.

"I don't know, but she's unconscious," Larry said.

"I bet she didn't take her shot," Milo said, hurrying to the kitchen. He took a small bottle from the refrigerator and returned to the room where Larry was still holding the receiver.

"I'm calling an ambulance," Larry said.

"That's not necessary," Milo said. "She just needs her shot." He held up the bottle. It was a medicine bottle, but the label was smeared and unreadable. "She keeps the whatchamacallits in that drawer." He took a disposable syringe from the drawer and handed it to Larry. "Here. You do it."

Larry shook his head. "No," he said without explaining further. He did not take the syringe.

"It's easy," Milo said. "I did it last year when this happened. Mrs. Thompson said you have lots of experience from the hospital, so you do it."

"I'm a licensed practical nurse," Larry stated.

The man thrust the syringe at Larry. "Then do it!" he shouted angrily. "She might die."

At that moment Larry's call went through. He said there was an emergency and requested that an ambulance be sent immediately. Larry made Mrs. Thompson as comfortable as possible and waited. He monitored her breathing and pulse from time to time. Milo Davis glared at him but didn't say another word. He also didn't administer the medication in the bottle.

When the ambulance was gone, Milo finally spoke. "How dare you call yourself a nurse if you'll risk an old woman's life like that?" he snapped, brandishing the syringe like an accusing finger at Larry. "You're not a good neighbor, and you're certainly not a Good Samaritan. I don't know what you call yourself." With that he stalked out of the apartment.

Larry picked up the bottle and looked at the label. It was unreadable, but an expiration date was still legible. The date was over 2 years old. He held the bottle to the light. A suspiciously cloudy mass swirled inside the bottle.

After the ambulance took Mrs. Thompson to the hospital, Larry smiled as he remembered what Milo had said. "What I call myself is a good neighbor, a Good Samaritan, and a *very* good nurse," he said as if the man were still there. "And do you know why I'm a good nurse? I'll tell you. It's because I know what to do and when to do it, what I can do within the law, and when to ask for help."

Contemporary practical/vocational nursing is an active process in which you will interact with your patients to provide care in a one-to-one relationship that is based on their trust and your competency. Your duty is to do good and to avoid harm in accordance with the law.

Laws are rules of conduct derived from cultural values, moral practices, and ethical beliefs. In a democracy, they are made and enforced by the authority of the group to whom they apply.

Good Samaritan Statutes

The story of the Good Samaritan tells of a man who was beaten and robbed and then left to die at the side of the road. People walking by ignored him. But one man, a Samaritan, did not. He dressed the injured man's wounds and took him to safe lodging, without being asked and without being paid. Today, *Good Samaritan laws* protect people from prosecution who voluntarily go to the aid of others in an emergency if the person providing emergency care did not act recklessly or did not intentionally harm the victim.

Good Samaritan laws have been passed by virtually every state. They vary from state to state, and you are responsible to find out what the statute in your state says. Generally such laws require that people who render aid are expected to act as any reasonable, prudent person would in that situation. Nurses and other health care practitioners are expected to render care equal to that of another practitioner with the same level of skill, training, and experience. The intention of Good Samaritan laws is to encourage the giving of emergency care outside the hospital or health care facility.

However, it is important to note that nobody, whether health care practitioner or lay person, is obligated by law to give emergency care outside the health care setting. To act or not is an ethical decision you must make when faced with an emergency situation in a noninstitutional setting.

Sources of Laws

Laws come from two general sources. The first source is the government (either federal, state, or local), and laws from this source are termed "public laws." Public laws include laws based on the Constitution of the United States, the constitution of an individual state, or the constitution of a subdivision within a state. Federal laws are based on the U.S. Constitution and its amendments. State constitutional laws, among other things, identify the legal relationship between the state and its counties, townships, boroughs, municipalities, and villages. Municipal (city) constitutional law prescribes the form of government through which the city will operate and conduct its business.

Another type of public law creates administrative agencies that have the power to make and enforce rules and regulations. Nurse practice acts are laws that are passed by state governments to control the practice of nursing in that state. The state government appoints, elects, or selects members of a committee, usually called the state board of nursing, to interpret and enforce the law. Nurse practice acts and state boards of nursing will be discussed in more detail later in this chapter.

The last type of public law, criminal law, deals with offenses against the welfare or safety of the public. Criminal law includes minor offenses, misdemeanors, and felonies. A misdemeanor applies to offenses that do not qualify as felonies. A conviction for a felony makes a person liable for the death sentence or for a life sentence in a federal or state prison. A felony is a more serious crime than a misdemeanor. The federal government determines what constitutes a federal crime, and each state has the power to determine what it considers a crime.

The second source of law is called private law. The focus of private law is the enforcement of rights, duties, and other legal relations between private citizens. Laws related to enforcing contracts and laws related to torts, which are legal wrongs not included under contract law, are two divisions of private laws that are of particular interest to nurses.

Table 10-1 summarizes the major divisions within public law and private law. The examples included in this table are intended to help you understand the differences between public law and private law.

Nursing Practice and the Law

The basic law governing your practice as a practical/vocational nurse is the nurse practice act (a constitutional law) that was passed by your state legislature. You will recall that after a bill is passed, it becomes law, and that law is known as an act. A nurse practice act usually defines the legal functions, powers, and duties of the state board of nursing. It also identifies the membership of the board and how people become board members. A nurse practice act also defines terms such as "nursing" and the duties of the nurse practitioner, registered nurse, and practical or vocational nurse. The laws governing licensure and legal titles are also included in nurse practice acts. Any changes in the nurse practice act must be made through the state legislature and must follow the same process as any other proposed law.

Nurse practice acts are administered by state boards of nursing or committees with a similar title. Members of the state board of nursing are registered nurses, practical/vocational nurses, consumers, and others interested in the health and welfare of the citizens of the state. Such a board is usually appointed by the governor of the state, and the majority of its

Table 10-1.
Sources of Law

Public Law (also known as statutory law)

Constitutional Law
  Federal government (the U.S. Constitution and the Amendments)
  State government (the constitution of a state: many similarities to the U.S. Constitution)
  Local government (the constitution or similarly titled document that identifies the political
    structure and social responsibilities of local governing bodies)
Administrative Law
  Federal (Occupational Safety and Health Administration)
  State (state boards of nursing)
  Local (city department of licenses and inspection)
Criminal Law
  Federal (transporting drugs between states)
  State (murder of a citizen of the state)
  Local (violation of a parking law)

Private Law (also known as civil or common law)

Contract Law (implied, oral, written)
  Written contracts (such as school loans)
  Verbal contracts ("I will babysit for you on Saturday from 7 P.M. to 1 A.M.)
Law of Torts (legal wrong not included under contract laws)
  Negligence
  False imprisonment
  Confidentiality
  Defamation of character
  Consent
  Assault and battery
  Fraud

---

members are registered nurses. Other members may include consumer representatives and licensed practical/vocational nurses. The board is headed by a salaried executive director, usually a registered nurse, who, with a paid staff, manages daily matters related to nursing in that state.

State boards have legal authority to interpret, implement, and enforce the law governing nursing practice, nursing education, and licensure. Disciplinary hearings for licensees and prosecution of violations of nurse practice acts are conducted by the boards.

Keep in mind that the law of the state in which you practice nursing is the law that applies to you and that ignorance of the law is not an excuse for illegal acts. You must know the law and practice within it, and you are held responsible for your own acts as a nurse.

Responsibility

Responsibility is the condition of being accountable for your actions. Whether you are a student or an employee, many of your responsibilities will be well defined in the written or verbal contract you enter into with your school or employer. But because nurses have a relationship with patients that includes touching, treating, collecting information, and providing personal services, you will have a number of other responsibilities that are not written and are not easily defined. These are responsibilities that come with the job.

You are legally obligated by the nurse practice act and the public and private laws of your state to provide a certain standard of care and to practice nursing within the law. In addition, the National Federation of Licensed Practical Nurses (NFLPN) and the National Association for Practical Nurse Education and Service (NAPNES) standards (Appendixes D and E), as well as employer guidelines, determine what your job responsibilities are. The level of care you are expected to give is to be equal to the care reasonably expected from other nurses with similar training and experience in a similar situation.

Liability

As stated, accepting responsibility for one's actions means that the individual who commits an act is the one who must explain the act and accept any consequences that follow. A student who borrows a library book and then loses it is responsible for what happened to the book and accountable for its replacement.

Liability is the legal obligation a person has to make good for the loss of, or damage to, something for which he is responsible. In the case of the library book, the student who lost it would be liable (obligated) to replace or pay for it.

A person is always responsible and liable for his actions. As a nurse, you are legally responsible for the care you give or neglect to give your patients, as well as for your professional and personal conduct. Your best protection against charges regarding the performance of your duties, whether a legal action or a personal criticism, is to carry out your duties at or above the standards expected from someone with your education, ability, and experience. Even then, it is possible that a charge could be made against you, particularly in a social climate that fosters lawsuits.

Legal Relationships Between the Employer and the Employee

The legal relationship between the employer and the employee is fairly well defined. The employer has the right to direct and control the performance of work. An employee is a person who accepts wages as a result of the service he provides to the employer.

A legal term, *respondeat superior,* is used to describe the legal responsibility of an employer for the acts of his employee. In other words, both the nurse who injures a patient and the nurse's employer can be held liable for the nurse's acts.

To protect themselves and their employees from potential legal problems, employers and institutions develop guidelines governing their operations. These guidelines are not laws; they are policies that state what action is expected in specific situations. They are often more explicit than laws in that they provide detailed procedures and clear directions. Thus it is imperative that you become thoroughly familiar with these guidelines.

Because institutional and employer guidelines must reflect current conditions to be effective, they are changed periodically. Your duties will put you in daily contact with your employer's policies and procedures. You will be in an excellent position to know whether these guidelines are meeting the needs they were written for and to suggest changes when they are not.

Contracts

A contract is an agreement between two or more parties. Contracts are written or verbal promises in which something of value is exchanged. A verbal agreement to meet a friend is a social obligation and is not classified as a contract. A nurse who accepts employment offered either by an institution, a health care provider, or a patient is entering into a contract. The value exchanged in this type of contract is money (from the employer) for the services (nursing).

When entering into an employment contract, you should have a written agreement that defines hours and wages, the length of the contract, fringe benefits, vacation periods and lengths, length of sick leave, hours of work each week, insurance coverage, and job responsibilities expected by the employer. The employer, in turn, expects you to provide the services for which you will receive these benefits. These services are often understood to be those which are expected of anyone with the same education and license that you have.

"Breach of contract" is the term used to describe the failure of one of the parties to a contract to fulfill his obligations under the contract. Breach-of-contract suits against nurses are most often suits in which damages are claimed. Damages are awarded to the complaining person if it can be shown that the plaintiff (complaining person) has suffered a financial loss. For example, suppose you agree to provide practical/vocational nursing services to one patient for 8 hours for $80. If you do not keep this contract, and the patient has to employ a practical/vocational nurse for $90 for that 8-hour period, the patient (plaintiff) may have a cause to act against you.

Torts

A tort is an injury or wrong committed by one person against another. Nurses who provide nursing service frequently find themselves in situations where their behavior could result in a lawsuit claiming malpractice. "Malpractice" is the general term that describes the neglect of a physician or nurse to apply his education and skills, in caring for a patient, that other physicians or nurses customarily apply in caring for similar patients in similar circumstances.

Negligence

Negligence is a legal wrong that does not fit into the category of contracts under private law. Negligence includes professional misconduct, lack of skill in performing duties, and illegal or immoral conduct. If an act is so atrocious and human life has been endangered or even lost, the action is usually called gross negligence, and a charge against the person may be filed in criminal courts and criminal charges brought against the defendant. Crimes related to nurses will be discussed in more detail later in the chapter.

Negligence also includes errors of omission and errors of commission. For negligence to be claimed, the nurse must have failed to do something that any reasonable and prudent nurse would have done in the same situation. In addition, some injury must result from the nurse's failure to act. Typical acts of negligence by nurses include failure to protect patients from burns caused by water bottles, bath water, or compresses, failure to ensure that bed rails are in place so that patients do not fall, failure to make sure that wrong dosages or medications are not given, and failure to properly identify patients before performing treatments.

Nurses commit acts of gross negligence when they perform duties beyond their education, experience, or legally defined limits. For example, if you administer a prescription medication without a physician's order and the patient dies as a result of your action, you may be guilty of gross negligence. You may be tried under private laws (tort) as well as under criminal law. Nurses must perform their duties as any ordinary, reasonable, and prudent nurse would in similar circumstances. And prudent nurses do not administer prescription medications without a physician's order.

False Imprisonment

A nurse cannot confine or restrict a patient to a place against his will except in situations specified by law (for example, when a physician orders it, or in an emergency situation where the patient might harm himself or others). Physical or verbal constraint without the consent of the patient or appropriate authority is false imprisonment.

"Constraint" means the prevention of free movement by any means. To keep a patient confined anywhere by threat of reprisal ("I'll take away your television privileges"), by removing his clothes, or by actual physical constraint (tying a patient to his bed) can all be acts of false imprisonment unless appropriate measures are followed, even when done in the patient's best interest.

Always record your efforts to inform a patient why he should be restricted. If he refuses, notify your instructor.

Patients with psychiatric problems are more likely to bring charges of false imprisonment, but any patient might do so, particularly if confused or uninformed of the reason he is being constrained.

Confidentiality

Even though the principle of confidentiality in the nurse-patient relationship has not been clearly settled in the courts and is not recognized in some states, you are ethically obligated to treat information about your patients as confidential. Your intimate relationship with the lives of your patients gives you access to matters and information that in ordinary circumstances would be private. This information is privileged and should be treated as such.

Unless the information you have suggests that harm would come to the patient or to others if it is withheld, you should respect its private nature. Normal exchanges of information with your supervisor and other members of the patient's health care team in the performance of your duties are not subject to this restraint. However, discussing a patient in public— whether confidential information is mentioned or not—may place a nurse in danger of being accused of breaking the principle of confidentiality. So-called "shoptalk" (idly discussing or gossiping about patients with co-workers and others) should be avoided for this reason alone.

The release of information to anyone other than those persons directly associated with caring for the patient, without his permission, is a violation of the patient's right to privacy. It is generally outside the nurse's responsibility to provide information about patients to anyone, including the police, media, relatives, or visitors. Familiarize yourself with your program's, and later your employer's, standards on how patient information is to be handled and follow them.

Defamation of Character

Making false or malicious (intentionally harmful) statements to someone that hurt another person's character or reputation is defamation, or defamation of character. When the statements are made orally, they constitute slander; when written, they are called libel. Both are violations of law and ethics, and they can be causes for lawsuits.

You can protect yourself against accusations of slander or libel by restricting your verbal or written comments about patients—or anyone else—to nonjudgmental, objective statements of fact. Limit discussion about patients to the appropriate time and place, and make statements in terms that can be documented. Avoid idle comments and gossip ("shoptalk"), and when charting, limit your written remarks to accurate, impartial statements.

Failure to Obtain Informed Consent

A fundamental right of patients is to make decisions regarding their own medical care. This right means that patients can accept or reject medical treatment. A patient who accepts medical treatment is said to give consent. For consent to be legal, it must be both voluntary, meaning that it is freely given, and informed, meaning that the patient clearly understands his alternatives.

Voluntary, informed consent by the patient to medical treatment is required by law. The right to informed consent is also specified in the AHA's "Patient's Bill of Rights" (see Appendix H). Consent is obtained from a patient either verbally or in writing, with written consent preferred. The physician is responsible for getting a patient's consent for certain procedures; the nurse is responsible for getting a patient's consent for nursing care.

If a patient seems unclear or poorly informed about his treatment, tell your instructor, so that the patient's physician or nursing team leader can provide additional clarification.

Once given, consent can be withdrawn by the patient, and withdrawal of consent may occur at the most unexpected times.

Technically, you should ask for and receive consent from your patients before administering every nursing procedure. This isn't as cumbersome as it sounds, because patients are expected to have a reasonable awareness of the nature of nursing care. Nevertheless, you should always inform your patients about what you are doing and ask their permission to do it. The request and the response don't have to be direct; they can be implied. For example, if you tell a patient you are there to bathe him and the patient says, "Yes, I'm ready for a bath," or words to that effect, he is giving direct consent. If he does not say anything, but nods or otherwise indicates by his actions that he is ready for a bath, he is giving implied consent. In both cases you have his consent to act. Conversely, if he says, "No bath today," or shakes his head, he is denying consent.

Obtaining direct or implied consent is always easier when the patient understands what is going on and why. Explain beforehand what you are doing and why it's necessary so that your patient can make an informed decision.

Consent for providing care for minors is obtained from the minor's parent or legal guardian. It's a good idea to get the minor's consent as well, whenever possible. If care has been authorized by a legal guardian and a minor refuses it, inform your instructor before proceeding with treatment or before withholding it. Consent for providing care for mentally incompetent patients must also come from a legal guardian.

In some instances a person may be unable to make an informed decision but is not legally incompetent. Intoxicated, unconscious, or confused patients are examples. It is not your responsibility to determine by whose authority consent can be given in such cases, but it's wise to know what the laws in your state are and what specific policy your employer or institution has regarding it.

Assault and Battery

One of the most common acts of nursing care, touching a patient, requires the patient's consent, whether the reason for touching is in his best interest or not. When direct or implied consent is not given, the potential for a charge of *battery*—touching another person without permission—is possible.

Permission to touch in a nursing care situation is generally implied, but you should always inform your patients about what you are doing. If permission to touch is refused, and explaining to the patient the reason that you need to touch him fails to change his mind, inform your instructor. Don't continue with the procedure.

Assault is the threat to touch without permission. A charge of assault can be brought even if the threat could not be carried out but the patient fears that it could. For example, telling a patient to take a prescribed medication or be faced with getting it by injection may get the patient to do as asked, but a charge of assault could be lodged.

Fraud

Fraud is intentional deception to prevent a person from receiving what is lawfully his. In a health care setting, a patient who has been charged for a service that was not performed has been defrauded. A nurse who falsely tells a patient that a medication has no side effects, so that the patient will take it could be charged with fraud. It would be fraudulent to change a chart to cover up an error that, if discovered, could result in an action against the person who made the entry.

Malpractice Claims

Charges of poor care, patient harm, and patient dissatisfaction do not usually end in malpractice claims and lawsuits. But when they do, they are often influenced by factors you should recognize.

The public is increasingly sensitive to the real or imagined impersonality of the American health care system. When health care is seen as big and profitable business, patients within the system are more apt to enter a lawsuit for an alleged wrong. The fact that health care employers and practitioners carry liability insurance is used by people to justify claims against them. This is especially true of large claims against health care providers, since many people believe that "insurance companies pay them anyway, and they [the insurance companies] can afford it." Also, frequent news stories of enormous judgments awarded in lawsuits may encourage some patients to initiate one to offset high medical care costs or even to solve financial woes.

Some patients are more likely to claim malpractice and bring a lawsuit than others. Called "suit prone," they are quick to sue for damages whether or not the damages are real or the suit is justified. Some of the traits they exhibit include high levels of criticism, faultfinding, hostility, uncooperativeness, and sensitivity to being offended. Success in earlier lawsuits in which they have been awarded damages (payment) may also encourage some patients to try again.

Use moderation when dealing with such patients. Work to meet their needs, rather than turn defensive or confrontational. Nurses who fail to respond to their patients' needs, who are insensitive and uncaring, or who exceed their own limits in providing care may encourage a lawsuit.

Not all malpractice claims can be prevented, but many can be discouraged by strict personal and institutional adherence to high standards of health care. Some general directions related to patient charts, wills, and gifts may help you avoid claims of malpractice.

Patient Charts

Your patient's chart is a legal record of his hospitalization. The importance of the accuracy of the chart, not only as an ongoing record of events, but as a lasting document that can be referred to later if the need arises, cannot be overstated. The care by which a chart is kept protects the patient during his stay and can be used to protect those who administered his care in the event of a lawsuit later. In both cases the level of protection is determined by how well the chart is kept. Anything that is not recorded on a patient's chart is presumed not to have happened, even if it did.

Charts and charting procedures will be described to you by your instructor. Later, when you are employed, you will find that charts vary from one institution to another. Procedures may also differ. Learn what is required and conform to that. Employers will expect you to be familiar with the charting process, but they will also recognize your need for time to learn the specifics of their system.

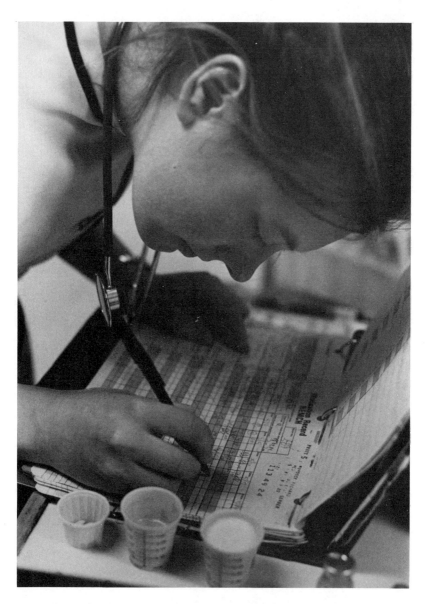

Patient charts are legal records of medical and nursing care. (© Richard Wood, Taurus Photos.)

Be consistent when charting and use only agency-approved abbreviations and charting correction procedures, so that any given entry always means the same thing whenever it is written and so that errors will always be corrected properly.

Wills

A will is a legal statement of a person's wishes regarding the disposition of his property after death. There may be times when patients ask you to help them prepare their wills. You should not accept the responsibility but should refer the matter to your instructor. An attorney is the appropriate person to help someone write a will, and the patient should be assisted to find one if he requests it.

On occasion, you may be asked to witness a patient's will. Not all institutions allow nurses to sign wills. Abide by the guidelines set by yours. If signing is permitted, because more than one witness will be required, sign a will only when the other witnesses and the person whose will it is are present. Be sure the act of signing is accurately entered on the patient's chart, with particular attention to the time and date of the signing.

Gifts

As a nurse, you should make it clear to patients and families that you do not accept gifts. It is legal to do so, but it is not ethical to accept gifts. And it is certainly not ethical to solicit them.

However, there may be times when a patient may wish to give personal possessions as gifts to various people, including members of the health care team. This may be out of gratitude for the care the patient has received or because he realizes that death is near. If the patient owns or has the right to dispose of the gift, and if the recipient accepts the gift, the act is valid within the law as long as the patient understands what he is doing and has not been coerced or deceived by anyone. Courteous refusal to accept the gift is the more appropriate response.

If a refusal is not accepted by the patient, particularly in times when the emotional climate is high, you should always protect yourself from any question about accepting a gift by having a witness present, informing your instructor or supervisor, and recording the patient's condition at the time.

Table 10-2 summarizes guidelines for avoiding malpractice claims.

Malpractice Insurance

Malpractice insurance for nurses is becoming increasingly important in a society that has become suit conscious.

Paying for the defense of a lawsuit and paying any judgment that might be rendered are beyond the ability of most people. To protect their

Table 10-2.
Guidelines for Avoiding Malpractice Claims

- Maintain a healthy self-awareness of your competence to practice.
- Avoid allowing what you do to become so routine and unthinking that you perform your duties automatically.
- Find out what your strengths and weaknesses are and deal with each according to its need.
- Capitalize on what you do well and seek to improve those areas that need help through education, experience, or guidance from others.
- Don't hesitate to ask for advice from competent advisers.
- Don't accept or perform duties that you are unsure of or for which you lack education, training, or experience.
- Evaluate assignments and establish priorities.
- Do not assume the role or duties of health care providers whose qualifications exceed yours.
- Don't "practice medicine" for friends and neighbors.
- Stay informed of your employer's procedures and policies.
- You have the right to refuse to do anything you are not qualified to do, that is unclear to you, or that is against stated policies, laws, nurse practice acts, and other legal restrictions.
- When you see a policy that is outdated, ineffective, or wrong, bring it to the attention of your instructor or appropriate authority so that the policy can be changed.
- Maintain accurate, legible, consistent, and complete records in strict accordance with your employer's policies.
- Continuously observe the safety rules and regulations set by your employer.
- Be aware that some practices in one's personal life—use of alcohol or drugs, for example—or other behavior that reflects poorly on one's character may be used against one in a malpractice suit.

employees and themselves against any legal and financial consequences that could arise from their provision of services, institutional employers carry liability insurance. However, because individuals are responsible for their actions, it is still possible for an employee—you as a nurse, for example—to be sued personally. This is true even in states where "charitable immunity"—the protection of nonprofit hospitals from legal liability—applies. A separate, personal liability insurance policy over and above your employer's policy is a wise investment that some would consider essential.

For your personal protection against claims against you, make certain your employer carries a policy of liability insurance that covers you. Find out the exact nature and limits of the coverage it gives you. Then, with a knowledgeable expert, determine what additional personal coverage you should carry and purchase a policy accordingly.

Crimes

A crime is an offense that is committed against the public welfare. You will recall that a tort is a legal wrong claimed by one person against another.

Therefore, if you commit a tort, the injured person is the one who prosecutes you. If you commit a crime, however, it is the state that seeks to prosecute you.

Criminal acts can be classified as minor offenses, misdemeanors, or felonies. Felonies are the most serious grade of criminal act and includes murder. Misdemeanors are less serious than felonies. An example of a misdemeanor is that of a nurse's practicing in a state with mandatory nursing licensure laws without a nursing license. Practicing without a license is a criminal offense punishable under public law.

Grossly negligent acts are considered crimes by many states. A nurse who restrains a patient against his will and without proper authorization may be charged with false imprisonment and prosecuted for committing a tort. However, if the same nurse became angry with the patient's behavior and restrained the patient with such force that his circulation was impaired for a prolonged period so that the patient's hand had to be amputated, the nurse would most likely be charged with a crime. To convict a nurse of a crime, the court would have to prove both a criminal act and a criminal intent.

In addition to grossly negligent acts, other crimes in which nurses may become directly or indirectly involved include situations related to the death of a patient, violations of federal and state narcotic and controlled substance laws, fraud related to falsifying patient bills, and robbery related to a patient's belongings.

In your nursing practice, you must practice within the law. You must be certain that your actions are based on your education, experience, standards of practice, and employer guidelines and not on emotional responses to sometimes difficult situations. You must think about what you are doing, why you are doing it, and whether a nurse with your similar education and experience would take the same or similar action as you intend to take.

Discussion Questions/Learning Activities

1. Read the Fourteenth Amendment to the Constitution of the United States. Do you find in this amendment the basis for any present laws?
2. Obtain a job description for licensed practical/vocational nurses from your affiliating agency. Analyze how clearly the duties of the LP/VN are written.
3. Read your malpractice insurance policy if you have one. What acts are included and what acts are excluded?

(Continued)

4. Ask your librarian to refer you to books that present summaries of malpractice suits. What similarities do you find in cases of negligence?
5. In addition to the suggestions presented in the chapter, what other actions by a nurse may reduce the possibility of a claim of malpractice?
6. Obtain and review the policy and procedures manual compiled by your affiliating agency. How do these documents define the standards of practice expected of this agency?
7. Imagine that you are driving to school and an automobile accident occurs in front of you. When you stop, you see that the driver of the car has hit his head on the windshield. What will you do and why?
8. Obtain a copy of the nurse practice act for your state. Analyze how these laws affect your practice of nursing.

References

Bernzweig EP: The Nurse's Liability for Malpractice: A Programmed Course. New York, McGraw-Hill, 1987.

Creighton H: Law Every Nurse Should Know. Philadelphia, WB Saunders, 1981.

Ford RD (ed): Nurses' Legal Handbook. Springhouse, PA, Springhouse, 1985.

Hemelt M, MacKert M: Dynamics of Law in Nursing and Health Care. East Norwalk, CT, Appleton & Lange, 1982.

Murchison IA: Legal Accountability in the Nursing Process. New York, Macmillan, 1982.

Northrop CC, Kelly MC: Legal Issues in Nursing. St. Louis, CV Mosby, 1987.

11 Effective Leadership, Management, and Membership

Objectives

When you complete this chapter, you should be able to:

Describe some of the personal qualities of an effective leader.

Outline the skills associated with managing patient care.

Identify skills that are related to managing the patient unit.

Describe some of the general responsibilities of the charge nurse for maintaining a safe environment.

Provide suggestions for communicating with supervisors, visitors, and physicians.

Explain the purpose of student organizations.

Name, and give the purposes of, the nursing organizations to which LP/VNs usually belong.

Describe the influence of the political process on health care.

The notice was posted where everyone in the program could see. It read:

Student Council Meeting
to elect officers, Friday at 3 P.M. in
Tully Hall

"Are you going?" Maria asked her new friend, Roz.

Roz shook her head. "I don't think so," she said. "I have to go home right after our last class."

"Mrs. Draper said they're going to elect officers," Maria said. Mrs. Draper was the program director.

Roz furrowed her brow.

"Don't you want to try?" Maria asked.

Roz made a face. "For student council officer?".

"Sure," Maria said. "Why not? You'd be good at it."

Roz laughed. "Now I know you're joking with me," she said.

But Maria was serious. "I'm not joking. You're a really good student, people like you, and, besides, we're going to have a student council one way or the other. It's up to us to decide what kind of council it's going to be. A good council can influence the whole class. And when a class looks good, people notice. Employers, for example."

Maria changed her voice as if to imitate a very serious personnel director. "Oh, you were in Mrs. Draper's program last year," she said. "I heard all about your class." Then she switched back to her own voice. "Don't you see? When a class has goals and works together on things to get them done, it, well, it brings them together and everybody benefits."

"I *do* know what you mean," Roz said brightly. "We had a prom committee like that in high school. They still talk about it because ours was the best prom anybody had ever seen."

Maria beamed. "That's the whole point," she said. "If we have a good student council, we can do the same thing. We can work together, get things done—come on, Roz, change your plans for Friday. Go to the meeting with me."

Roz opened the notebook she kept her schedule in. She thought for a moment; then she nodded. "Okay," she said. "I'll go." Then she laughed again. "But you know something? You should be a politician."

A sly smile crossed Maria's face. "I am," she said. She glanced down the hall. Two other students were talking together. "Come on," she said to Roz. "Let's make sure they're going to be there, too."

On the Monday after the Friday meeting, a new notice was posted on the bulletin board:

Notice to All Students
The following officers were elected at
Friday's student council meeting:
President—Maria Ortega
Vice-President—Roz Taylor

That year, Mrs. Draper's class was already known among area health care facilities as the group to look to for excellent nurses with outstanding leadership potential.

A number of trends over the years have contributed to changing the roles and responsibilities of the licensed practical/vocational nurse. The passage of Medicare and Medicaid legislation in 1965 and changes in accreditation standards for nursing homes and other long-term care facilities have created an overall rise in the demand for nursing service, which has resulted in an increasing use of LP/VNs as team leaders, charge nurses, or patient care managers. This relatively new responsibility for specialized practical/vocational nursing practice is reflected in the 1987 NFLPN "Nursing

Practice Standards for the Licensed Practical/Vocational Nurse" (Appendix D). The LP/VN who is considering specialized nursing practice is expected to have at least 1 year's experience at the staff level, have personal qualifications that contribute to successful performance of specialized nursing practice, and complete a program or course of study designed to prepare an LP/VN for specialization.

Although it is still very early in your career, now is the time to begin developing the leadership qualities, management skills, and organizational activities that will contribute to your advancement in practical/vocational nursing.

Leadership Qualities

An effective leader is much easier to recognize than to describe. From your own experiences, you can no doubt identify team leaders, charge nurses, and patient care managers who are effective leaders and others who are not. Becoming an effective leader doesn't happen naturally; it takes study, experience, and work to develop a number of personal qualities.

Now is the time, early in your career, to begin studying and practicing the personal and interpersonal qualities of an effective leader.

Effective leaders are emotionally mature. They do not have temper tantrums, pout, complain, or find fault. They do not speak loudly or joke inappropriately in the presence of patients or their visitors. The emotionally mature leader is even tempered, tolerant, and patient and maintains a businesslike atmosphere everywhere, especially in patient care areas.

An effective leader is open-minded—willing to listen to the suggestions of others. The open-minded leader looks for better methods and safer procedures and frequently asks for the opinions of others.

An effective leader is fair. This means that the leader does not allow personal friendships and favoritism to cloud relationships with staff. They respect each member of the nursing team and expect everyone to make a maximum contribution to patient care.

Effective leaders are consistent. They are consistent in enforcing the policies regulating the conduct of their staff. On rare occasions when an exception can be justified, the staff members are given an explanation of the exception.

Effective leaders are responsible. They accept responsibility for the actions of their staff members and, when indicated, defend those actions to their superiors. When a staff member is at fault, they try to help that person make positive adjustments rather than dismissing them from the team.

An effective leader has a strong character. After making a decision, the leader changes the decision only when it is clear that the original decision

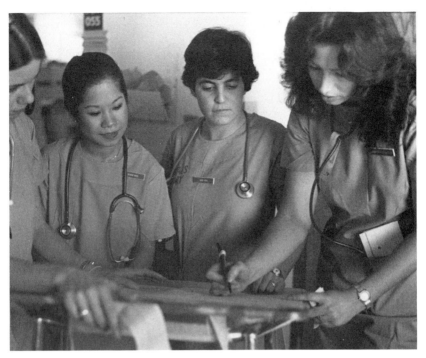

Becoming an effective leader requires study, experience, and the development of a number of personal and interpersonal qualities. (© Richard Wood, Taurus Photos.)

was a poor one. The leader with a strong character can admit to having made a poor decision and can offer a sincere apology to an individual who has been offended.

An effective leader has the ability to teach. The leader who has a desire to share knowledge and skills with others is well on the way to becoming a teacher. Patience, tolerance, and praise are qualities that enhance any teaching-learning situation.

An effective leader has developed excellent problem-solving abilities. The effective leader defines the problem, gathers the facts, analyzes the information, proposes several solutions and the consequences of each, makes a decision, and evaluates the effectiveness of the solution.

Effective leaders have excellent clinical skills. They recognize that they "set the standard" of care and serve as role models for the members of the staff. The effective leader offers workable suggestions and techniques to manage difficult nursing care situations.

Effective leaders are sensitive as well as objective. Although they enforce the rules and regulations of the employer and the unit, they are aware of the special needs and abilities of the people they are leading. They

---

Leadership Qualities

An effective leader is:

Emotionally mature	A problem solver
Open minded	Clinically proficient
Fair	Sensitive and objective
Consistent	Flexible
Responsible	Decisive
	One who profits from experience

---

interact with each member of their team as a unique human being with a vast array of personal needs and interests.

An effective leader often selects a role model who exemplifies the qualities of an effective leader. By observing the role model's personal and interpersonal relationships with staff members, the inexperienced leader can identify some of the personal qualities that contribute to effective leadership skills.

Effective leaders are flexible and match their style of leadership to the situation. During an emergency, the effective leader is decisive and gives direct orders to the team members. In the daily routine, the effective leader follows a fairly well established and consistent style of leadership. The effective leader who is making long-range plans may encourage suggestions from the members of the nursing team and incorporate their recommendations into the plan.

These are just a few of the personal qualities of an effective leader. These qualities may not come naturally, but you can develop them if you make an honest effort to incorporate them into your life and your nursing career. Do this by being aware of what they are, by observing them in yourself, by noting how they change as you practice them, and by making corrections when your actions do not produce the results you want. Learn from your mistakes.

It is important to know that leaders, no matter how much education or experience they have, make mistakes. Learning from your mistakes is a quality that will probably contribute most to your development as a leader. Being the leader of a patient care team is a tremendous responsibility but one that can provide equally tremendous rewards. The box above summarizes the qualities of an effective leader.

In addition to the leadership role, the team leader, charge nurse, or patient care manager must also have effective skills in management.

Management Skills

Management is the coordination of activities associated with providing patient care and delivering nursing services. Being a manager of a patient unit is a responsible position. Managers must have, in addition to leadership skills, skills in planning, organizing, and directing the work of others.

Managing Patient Care

The primary responsibility of a nurse manager (team leader, charge nurse, or patient care manager) is to direct patient care on a day-to-day basis. Other functions of the manager include ordering supplies and equipment, maintaining a safe environment, and communicating with other departments and with supervisors, physicians, and visitors.

Directing day-to-day patient care includes assessing staff capabilities, diagnosing patient needs for nursing care, planning for patient care, implementing the assignment, and evaluating the performance.

Assessing Staff Capabilities

The first step in directing patient care is assessment. You will need to assess the educational preparation of staff members, their experience, and the functions they are permitted to perform. (These functions are defined by the laws of your state and are also outlined in job descriptions developed by employers.)

Diagnosing Patient Needs for Nursing Care

The second step in directing patient care is to diagnose the particular nursing care needs of the patients on your unit. Does the patient need the skills that can be provided only by an LP/VN, or can a nursing assistant meet patient needs? At this point, you might also consider the personality of the patient. Although all nursing staff members should be able to meet the needs of any patient on your unit, it sometimes improves communication between the patient and the nurse when personalities are well matched.

Planning for Patient Care

The third step in directing patient care is to plan for patient care. This plan is generally communicated through a written assignment sheet or assignment board. The assignment sheet includes the name of the staff members, their break and meal times, the names and room numbers of the patients to whom they are assigned, and any other general duties the staff members are expected to complete during their time on duty.

Implementing Assignments

The fourth step in directing patient care is to post the written assignment sheet. The assignment sheet must be completed and available to the staff within 15 to 30 minutes of the beginning of the shift so that staff members can determine their priorities and organize their work for the day. Verbal directions along with the written assignments can avoid confusion and misunderstanding between the staff members and the leader.

On occasion, it may be necessary to change an assignment. When this happens, the manager must not only make the change on the written assignment sheet but must also verbally tell the staff member of the change. An effective leader would also explain why the change was necessary and acknowledge the effect that the change may have on the staff member.

Evaluating Performance

The fifth step in directing patient care is to evaluate the performance of your nursing staff. You might ask yourself the following evaluation questions: Do the patients have any comments on their nursing care? Are the assignments appropriate for the team members as well as the patients? Are assignments being completed on time? Are the break and meal times being followed? What changes would improve patient care?

If you find it necessary to discuss poor performance with a staff member, do so in a private place. Try to determine the cause of the poor performance, and if the team member is lacking the necessary knowledge or skills, provide the information that will help improve performance. Otherwise, suggest that a certain quality of patient care is expected and that you expect everyone to provide that quality.

If a staff member is behaving in a manner that is unsafe and inappropriate, discretely move the person away from patients and visitors and either call or have someone call for assistance from your supervisor. This difficult situation requires tact and sensitivity on the part of the leader and manager of the patient care unit.

In summary, these steps will help you plan, organized, and direct patient care on your nursing unit.

As you evaluate the performance of your staff and the quality of nursing care each day, you also collect information that will assist you when you begin the same process the next day. Experience can provide valuable lessons in developing skills that contribute to quality patient care.

Managing the Unit

In addition to managing patient care, the team leader, charge nurse, or patient care manager has many other functions that contribute indirectly to patient care. These functions are related to the operation of the patient care unit.

Ordering Supplies and Equipment

Supplies and equipment that are essential for patient care must be available to your nursing staff. The responsibility for having the necessary supplies and equipment on the patient unit belongs to the manager of the unit. You may delegate (assign) this responsibility to a member of your staff. If you assign these responsibilities to a member of your staff, you must periodically check the work to be sure supplies and equipment are being ordered properly.

All supplies, including drugs, must be put away promptly. Storage spaces must be kept neat and orderly so that items needed in an emergency can be quickly located. Equipment must be kept clean and in working order. Requests to repair equipment must be followed until repairs are completed.

Maintaining a Safe Environment

The physical environment consists of the surroundings in which you work. As a manager, you are responsible for seeing to it that unsafe situations are corrected. Although not everything that needs fixing can be fixed immediately, certain measures can be taken to prevent further damage or even injury to people in that environment. You don't have to nag to be persistent.

Carelessness often contributes to injuries to both your patients and your staff. Keep clutter to a minimum and clean up spills immediately. Keep bedside cabinet doors and drawers closed when they are not in use. Be sure your staff members remove supplies and equipment from the bedside when a task or procedure is completed. Check that beds and bed rails function properly. Remove broken chairs, wheelchairs, and similar equipment from your unit to prevent accidental use. Require your staff to keep the medication room or medication cart locked when not in use. With experience, common sense, and a concern for the safety of your patients and staff, you will develop a habit of looking for situations that are unsafe. As the manager, you must accept personal responsibility for correcting these situations.

A fire in a health care facility is one of the most frightening things that can happen. Require your staff to know the location of fire extinguishers, how to check pressure gauges on fire extinguishers, and how to use them. Be sure they know how to sound an internal fire alarm and when to call the local fire department. Review evacuation procedures and discuss the possibility of having a mock fire drill with your nursing supervisor.

Managing Communication

As we learned in Chapter 2, good communication skills are essential in nursing. You will want to be sure you understand information that you are receiving, and you will want to be clear in information you are giving.

Communicating With Visitors

Visitors are important to your patients and provide a diversion from the long hours alone in the health care facility. Most visitors are considerate and do not discuss topics that will upset your patients. If the patient does become upset or anxious, you must tactfully ask the visitors to limit their conversations to more neutral subjects.

Use caution when giving information about a patient to a visitor or a member of the family. What you know about a patient's diagnosis, laboratory results, or plan of treatment is essentially confidential and not to be shared with anyone. You can tactfully suggest that these kinds of questions are best answered by the patient's physician.

You can discuss nursing concerns such as food likes and dislikes, ambulation, and sleep patterns with the patient's family. If at all possible, this should be done in the presence of the patient, and the patient should be included in the conversation.

On occasion, visitors may become disruptive to the unit. As the manager, you must make an attempt to elicit their cooperation in controlling the noise. If you are unsuccessful, you should immediately notify your nursing supervisor and ask for assistance.

Communicating With Supervisors

Your relationships with your nursing supervisors can be both positive and beneficial to you. It is important to recognize that your nursing supervisor is ultimately responsible for the quality of nursing care that you and your staff provide. You should view your supervisor as a resource person to whom you can go for advice and assistance in managing your patient unit.

To maintain a good working relationship with your nursing supervisor, you must keep the supervisor informed of problems or incidents that occur on your unit. Problems that may seem small and insignificant to you may turn out to be major problems to the institution. You must also report your errors and the errors of your staff to your supervisor and complete a written description of any incident that occurs on your unit.

When you communicate with your nursing supervisor, it is important to clearly, concisely, and objectively present the facts of the situation. It is unfair to the supervisor, who will probably have to make a decision related to a situation, to present only what you want the supervisor to know.

Your supervisor is, like you, in a management position. Just as your subordinates will not always like or understand all your decisions, you will not like or understand all the decisions of your supervisor. You must contribute to developing a relationship with your supervisor that is positive and productive, not negative and destructive.

Communicating With Physicians

Communicating with the physician or primary care provider is an essential part of management in nursing. As in communicating with your supervisor, you should keep the physician informed of changes in the condition of his patient. You must be able to clearly and concisely describe the facts you are reporting.

If a physician's treatment or medication order is unclear or questionable, it must be verified with the physician. You are not expected to blindly follow orders that you believe could be harmful to your patients. It is important to use tact and good communication skills when requesting verification from the physician.

You, through your staff, are in a position to provide valuable information about patients to their physicians. Nurses spend a great deal of time with patients and consequently have information that may influence the methods a physician may choose in treating patients. Sharing that information through verbal communications with physicians can make an enormous contribution to the total plan of care for the patients. Thus the team leader, charge nurse, or patient care manager must establish effective methods of communication with physicians.

In summary, leading and managing patient care is a tremendous responsibility, but with that responsibility can come equally tremendous rewards. You can enjoy the satisfaction that comes from working with your staff, your supervisor, and with physicians to provide the quality of nursing care that you alone could never achieve.

Organizations

Organizations are social groups organized for a specific purpose. You can probably think of many examples of organizations that were formed for a specific purpose.

Organizations require bylaws and procedural rules (rules of order) if their stated purpose is to be met. Meetings also follow established procedures or run the risk of accomplishing nothing. Meetings generally follow recognized rules of order, the most familiar being *Robert's Rules of Order*. These rules define the duties and responsibilities of the officers and organize discussion, vote taking, and other procedures. Minutes, which are detailed notes of the business conducted in a meeting, become a permanent record of an organization's meetings.

Two types of organizations are important to you as a nursing student: student organizations and nursing organizations.

Student Organizations

Your nursing program may be an integral part of a larger institution, or it may be small and independent. The type, complexity, and size of its student government will reflect the nature of its affiliation. A program that is a part of a college, for example, must take into account the regulations that apply to living on campus, whereas a vocational school program with only day students does not. The bylaws of the student governments of each will be either complex or simple, according to the needs and purposes of the group.

A student council is the most common form of student organization. It is a group made up of student and faculty members who serve as representatives of the student body to the sponsoring organization. Student members are elected by the student body. A faculty member elected by the student body serves as adviser to the student council.

The function of the student council is to make recommendations to the sponsoring organization on matters affecting the students. Such matters include the rules that govern students—their social, recreational, and extracurricular activities and student discipline. The council also serves as a disciplinary board for infractions of school regulations. The precise manner in which each council operates is set by its bylaws. Secure a copy of your student council's bylaws and read them, because they relate directly to your student life.

Involvement with your student council or government is an opportunity for you to have a voice in the daily affairs of your education and a chance to learn and exercise leadership skills. Involvement does not mean that one must be on the council. It means to participate with it as an active, interested member of a student body with a common goal. It can also mean volunteering to be on special committees.

Practical/vocational nursing students in programs sponsored by larger organizations may have an opportunity to join other student organizations. These other organizations may emphasize politics, photography, journalism, or drama, to name a few possibilities.

One student organization of particular interest to practical/vocational nursing students is Health Occupations Students of America (HOSA). HOSA is a national organization with state affiliations and local chapters in secondary and postsecondary schools that offer courses in the field of health care and related services.

The purpose of this organization, which held its constitutional convention in 1976, is to assist students in developing vocational understanding, an awareness of social intelligence, civic consciousness, and leadership skills. HOSA chapter members participate in local, state, and national competitions in health-related areas.

If your school does not have a HOSA chapter, you might want to ask your faculty to consider sponsoring this worthwhile activity. Details on how to begin your own chapter are available from the national HOSA office. See Appendix F for the address of the national HOSA office.

Alumni Associations

If your program or school has an alumni (graduates) association, you and your classmates will have the opportunity to join other graduates of your program or school after your own graduation. By joining and becoming active, you can keep in touch with one another and with the activities, programs, and progress of the school itself. Your experience will become valuable to those who follow you, just as the suggestions and help of those who have gone before you have benefited your own education.

Keeping in touch with your school and class can also provide you with access to continuing education programs, job opportunities, information on advances and changes in practical/vocational nursing, and other developments of special interest to you.

Nursing Organizations

Being active as a nurse and being active in nursing are not the same. Being active as a nurse means working as a nurse. To be active in nursing means participating in nursing organizations. Belonging to nursing organizations is important to your development as a practical/vocational nurse. The specific purpose of each organization is unique, but the intention in all such organizations is to benefit the membership.

Practical/Vocational Nursing Organizations

The two national organizations designed to meet the particular needs of the practical/vocational nurse are the National Federation of Licensed Practical Nurses (NFLPN) and the National Association for Practical Nurse Education and Service (NAPNES).

The NFLPN was founded in 1949, and membership is limited to licensed practical/vocational nurses and student practical/vocational nurses. The primary purpose of this organization is to promote the practice of practical nursing. NFLPN, through its organizational structure and membership, develops positions on the educational requirements for the practice of practical/vocational nursing, makes recommendations related to continuing education, defines ethical conduct, and outlines standards and scope of practical/vocational nursing practice, all of which are based on a clearly defined philosophy of practical/vocational nursing. In addition, the NFLPN attempts to influence legislation affecting the licensed practical/vocational nurse through national and state lobbying programs.

NAPNES was founded in 1941 to promote the special interests of practical/vocational nurses and to assist schools in developing educational programs. Membership is open to licensed practical/vocational nurses, practical/vocational nursing students, practical/vocational nursing school faculty and directors, and others who are interested in promoting the practice of practical/vocational nursing. The primary purpose of NAPNES is to promote an understanding of practical/vocational nursing and to develop continuing education opportunities for LP/VNs. NAPNES also develops positions on the education of practical/vocational nurses, defines ethical conduct, and publishes standards of nursing practice. The NAPNES official publication, the *Journal of Practical Nursing,* and a newsletter, *NAPNES Forum,* keep the members informed of organizational activities.

The future of practical/vocational nursing depends a great deal on the effectiveness of these two organizations. Since organizations are made up of people who share a common goal, it is important to your future as a licensed practical/vocational nurse that you actively participate in either one or both of these organizations. The address of both organizations is listed in Appendix F.

National League for Nursing

The National League for Nursing (NLN) was founded in 1952, and membership is open to anyone interested in promoting health care through nursing service. This national organization is primarily concerned with the education of nurses and improving the quality of health care. The official publication of the NLN is *Nursing and Health Care.*

The NLN is a large organization, and many of its activities are conducted through special divisions called councils. The Council of Practical Nursing Program (CPNP) is concerned with those issues that affect practical/ vocational nursing. The CPNP is the division of the NLN that accredits practical/vocational nursing education programs and provides continuing education opportunities for faculty and program directors. CPNP also promotes the interests of practical/vocational nursing within the NLN. Persons who are interested in joining the NLN can find the address in Appendix F.

Whichever organizations you choose to join, do so with the intention of being an active member. It can be an investment in a future that you can improve while at the same time helping others improve theirs. Remember, organizations depend on members, and the strength of the members will determine the strength of the organization.

Political Process

Health care in the next 10 to 20 years will be greatly influenced by local, state, and federal legislative action. As a member of the health care team and as a citizen of this country, you are now and will continue to be affected by these political decisions. For example, political efforts to control rising health care costs may affect your salary, political efforts to revise the Medicare system may make it necessary for you to care for an aging or ill parent in your home, health care services may be reduced as a result of political actions and your job may be eliminated, or political action establishing new health care services may increase your personal income taxes.

A a nurse, you are in a unique position to see the problems from the patient's point of view, the health care system's point of view, and a personal point of view. You will have opinions and recommendations that you will probably want to share with your legislators.

You can affect the political process in several ways. The best-known way is to vote. Learn the positions of candidates on various issues and vote for those who you think will serve the interests of the people.

Another way to affect the political process is to write to your legislator. Elected officials need and want to know your views and opinions. Examples of how to address envelopes and letters to state and national legislators are shown on p. 206.

Other ways of affecting the political process include lobbying, negotiating, and demonstrating. Lobbying activities are conducted by organizations on behalf of the members. For example, NFLPN and NAPNES frequently lobby for or against legislation affecting LP/VNs.

Negotiating is the art of persuasion. In the political process, much time and energy is spent negotiating with and between legislators. Promises are made, positions are changed, and decisions are eventually reached.

Demonstrations are techniques that sometimes influence the political process. Demonstrations call attention to a particular problem or issue in a dramatic fashion. Demonstrations, whether peaceful or violent, usually attract public attention. Demonstrations occur when the political process has been unresponsive to an issue of critical importance to a group of people.

Keeping informed of legislation that may affect you is not as difficult as it may seem. Your organizations, through their publications, keep members informed of current legislative events in both state and national governments. Your local newspaper and national news magazines are also sources of information on political issues.

If you become politically active as a nurse and a concerned citizen,

---

Forms of Address

State Senators   The Honorable _____
                                   Senate Chamber
                                   City, State, Zip Code
                                   Dear Senator _____ :

State Representatives   The Honorable _____
State Assembly Members   House of Representatives
                                   City, State, Zip Code
                                   Dear Mr./Mrs./Ms. _____ :

U.S. Senators   The Honorable _____
                                   United States Senate
                                   Senate Office Building
                                   Washington, DC 20515
                                   Dear Senator _____ :

U.S. Representatives   The Honorable _____
                                   House of Representatives
                                   House Office Building
                                   Washington, DC 20515
                                   Dear Mr./Mrs./Ms. _____ :

---

you should exercise care to avoid offending your employer. Your political convictions are personal, and you have no right to impose those convictions on your employer or your patients. For example, if you are actively involved in, and working to pass, pro-life legislation and your employer provides legal abortion services, it would be inappropriate for you to conduct political activities against your employer. Such conduct is unethical, and it puts both you and your employer in a difficult position.

The following fundamental tools are at your disposal to help you affect the processes that influence your life and career:

1. *Be informed.* Stay abreast of what is happening in nursing by reading newspapers and nursing journals, listening to news broadcasts, and watching television programs that address current issues in health care.
2. *Participate.* Join nursing organizations and activist groups and be active in their work.
3. *Vote.* Express your opinions, and vote for those you want to represent you in elections in your organizations, your community, your state, and your country.

4. *Communicate.* Let your representatives know your views through letters or meetings, and support their efforts to pass the laws and make the changes you favor.
5. *Influence Others.* Share your opinions with friends, colleagues, neighbors, and others.

To affect the political process, and therefore to affect decisions that have a direct bearing on your life, you must first realize that your opinion is important and that you have the right to express it. Also, even though an individual may seem insignificant in a large group, the group is made of nothing but individuals, and you are one of them.

Discussion Questions/Learning Activities

1. Think about someone you consider to be an effective leader. (This person does not necessarily have to be a nurse.) List the personal characteristics that you think make this person an effective leader.
2. Obtain the job or position descriptions for the members of the nursing team in your clinical affiliation. Analyze each for education, experience, and skills.
3. In addition to the responsibilities of the patient care manager discussed in this chapter, list some of the other duties that might be assigned to this person.
4. Suppose you are the charge nurse of a 20-bed patient in an extended care facility, and suppose one of the nursing assistants has not been coming back from her break on time. Outline what you would do and why.
5. While evaluating the quality of patient care, you notice that a bed rail is broken. What would you do first, and why?
6. During your clinical experience, listen carefully to a conversation between a nurse and the nurse's supervisor. Analyze the conversation for its effectiveness in communicating information, ideas, or both. Was the purpose of the conversation understood by both the supervisor and the nurse? Was mutual respect evident? Was the conclusion of the conversation satisfactory to both parties? Were any comments made by either party after the other left?
7. Review the bylaws of your student organization if you have one. Do they clearly state the purpose of the organizations and its rules of operation? Should the bylaws be revised?

(Continued)

8. Write to NFLPN and NAPNES and request copies of their by-laws and membership applications. Review this information and consider becoming a student member.
9. Select a problem related to health care that is currently being discussed in your state legislature. What are the issues? What are the positions of various special interest groups on the proposed legislation? Some topics that may be appropriate are catastrophic health insurance, regulating the cost of health insurance, laws affecting nursing practice (nurse practice acts), seat belt laws, and funding for nursing education.
10. After you investigate a political issue and reach a personal conclusion, write a letter to your congressperson, giving your reasons for urging support or nonsupport of the proposed legislation.

References

Bagwell M, Clements S: A Political Handbook for Health Professionals. Boston, Little Brown, 1985.

Bullough B, Bullough VL: History, Trends and Politics of Nursing. East Norwalk, CT, Appleton & Lange, 1984.

Health Care Education Staff. Group Leadership Skills. St. Louis, CV Mosby, 1986.

Holle ML, Blatchley ME: Introduction to Leadership and Management in Nursing. Boston, Jones and Bartlett, 1987.

Jameson DB: Leadership Handbook. New Castle, PA, Author (R.D. No. 4, Box 330), 1978.

Kron T: The Management of Patient Care: Putting Leadership Skills to Work. Philadelphia, WB Saunders, 1981.

Robert HM: The Scott, Foresman Robert's Rules of Order; newly revised. Glenview, IL, Scott, Foresman, 1981.

Sullivan EJ, Decker PJ: Effective Management in Nursing. Menlo Park, CA, Addison-Wesley, 1985.

Beginning Your Nursing Career

12

Objectives

When you complete this chapter, you should be able to:

Compile a list of places, other than hospitals and nursing homes, where an LP/VN could be employed.

Describe some of the techniques to ease the transition from student to employee.

Explain the value of a self-assessment before making a decision on what type of nursing position to apply for.

List several sources of information on available nursing positions.

Prepare a chart that includes areas that should be considered when evaluating positions.

Write a letter of application.

Prepare a personal resume.

Write a letter of resignation.

Compare the advantages and disadvantages of union membership.

Explain the purpose of the grievance process.

Define the term "burnout."

"This is our last class together. Before you leave, I'd like to say a few things that I hope you'll remember. I've enjoyed being your instructor for almost a year now. But I'm not speaking as your instructor today. What I have to say is coming from the heart of someone who cares about nursing and cares about each one of you.

"When I became a nurse, the 'field' was more like a small garden. Nursing was basic in those days, in the subjects we studied and in the job opportunities that were available. The world seemed like a much smaller place. There certainly were fewer people. 'Burnout' wasn't a word yet, and if 'gerontology,' 'substance abuse,' and 'hospice care' were, none of us had ever heard of them. But that doesn't mean some of us weren't ready for those and other words when they came. Those who weren't ready—and many of my classmates weren't, I'm sorry to say—have been left behind. And that's the 'message' in what I want to say to you today.

"There's no way that we—all of us on the staff here—could fully prepare you for the many choices you will be facing. There are simply too many. You've been busy enough learning what we could teach you—weren't you? The other things you will have to know—the choices you will be making—are going to be up to you. Once you graduate, you'll be on your own. Oh, we'd love for you to come back anytime, and you know you're always welcome. But out there, out in the world of nursing practice, you won't have someone to remind you to finish an assignment, to practice a procedure until perfect, or to read up on something you're uncertain of. Those things and many more will be expected from you—including things you haven't even heard of yet, just as my class hadn't heard of 'gerontology.'

"Now, just for a moment, let me pretend I'm one of you. This is what I would say: 'But, Mrs. Fuller, if we haven't heard of something, how are we supposed to know what to do?'" Yes, it sounds funny, but isn't that what you were thinking? I thought so. So listen now to the answer.

"Nursing is dynamic, growing, and ever expanding. It will never again be what it is today, and what it becomes tomorrow will also change. Nursing moves into the future automatically. Nurses do not. I'll say that again. Nurses do not *automatically* keep up with nursing. Nurses move into the future by listening, watching, and preparing for it.

"All of you are ready for graduation because you have prepared for it, day by day, for almost a year. Those of you who will be in nursing's future have to begin preparing for it, day by day, starting today.

"Thank you, class. You've been wonderful."

Today's newly graduated practical/vocational nurse has options undreamed of by nurses who completed their programs as late as the 1970s. Today's LP/VN can earn a good salary, enjoy excellent insurance benefits, receive tuition assistance, have flexible work schedules, and find employment in a variety of health care facilities.

Choosing from among these many options requires thoughtful preparation on your part. Knowing what career opportunities are available can help you in planning your nursing career.

Career Opportunities in Nursing

Just as you probably evaluated your educational options before you chose your nursing school, you must also evaluate your employment options. Selecting your first nursing position will be an important decision and one that should be made very carefully.

The employment opportunities for licensed practical/vocational nurses extend beyond those provided by hospitals and nursing homes. As private businesses and government agencies respond to the growing needs of a complex society, more areas where nursing care is needed are opening.

You have an opportunity to select the type of nursing that best meets your personal interests, needs, and capabilities.

Hospital Nursing

More nursing care is provided in hospitals than in any other health care setting because of the comprehensive services hospitals offer. Whether in emergency rooms, recovery rooms, intensive care units, pediatric units, or other centers for specialized inpatient and outpatient care, every facet of nursing is practiced on a daily basis in hospitals. Opportunities for a variety of experience for nurses in hospitals are therefore great.

The hospital nurse is an important part of a large and complex health care delivery team that includes physicians, nurses, administrative staff, social workers, laboratory personnel, and many others. The nurse's role in caring for the patient is especially important, because the nurse is usually the person who spends extended time at the bedside.

The exact nature of a nurse's work in a hospital is set by the institution's overall operating policies and philosophy. They are spelled out in detail in job descriptions. Each nurse is responsible for learning the job description and becoming familiar with the job descriptions of other staff members, including registered nurses, nurse's aides, technicians, orderlies, and attendants.

Hospital work schedules are generally set in three 8½-hour shifts: day (7 A.M. to 3:30 P.M.), afternoon (3 P.M. to 11:30 P.M.), and night (11 P.M. to 7:30 A.M.). Shift, weekend, and holiday rotations, time off, and other scheduling procedures are set by the institution. Scheduling may vary from one institution to another to accommodate staffing needs and the personal needs of employees.

Hospital nursing offers a variety of work experience, different kinds of patients, diverse nursing and medical situations, and often, abundant opportunity for career advancement.

Community and Public Health Nursing

A very different nursing setting is experienced by nurses who work in community or public health care. There, nursing is provided for the patient under the administration of established health care programs. These programs are operated and funded by voluntary agencies or local, state, or federal government agencies.

Nurses employed by public health programs may work inside community health centers with patients who come to the center, or they may work outside the center, traveling to the patient's home to give care there. The nursing staff of a city department of health clinic, for example, may

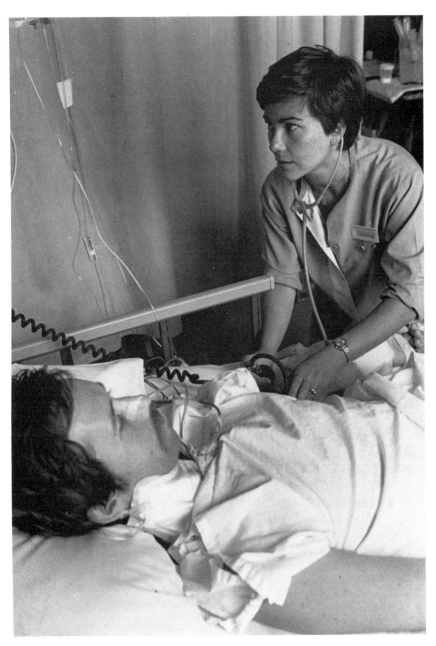

Employment opportunities for licensed practical/vocational nurses continue to expand.
(© Richard Wood, Taurus Photos.)

provide in-clinic immunizations, prenatal care and counseling, and other services to clients who visit the clinic, or they may give the same service at the client's residence.

The licensed practical/vocational nurse in a public health program will work under the direction of a registered nurse or other qualified supervisor. Among the qualifications for this work is the ability to work independently and responsibly when away from the health center.

Office Nursing

An especially challenging opportunity for a licensed practical/vocational nurse is that of the office nurse. As the employee of a physician, dentist, or other health practitioner, the nurse in an office may be responsible for a variety of duties that can include those of receptionist, secretary, lab assistant, bookkeeper, and supply clerk, plus the nursing skills for which licensure has been granted.

Flexibility, adaptability, and self-direction are assets for the office nurse, who may be required to perform preliminary patient examinations and routine treatments, oversee a waiting room full of patients, assist with treatments, schedule appointments, and collect payment at the end of a patient's visit.

Offices may be large or small, with a staff that matches, so responsibilities may be in the hands of a single nurse, shared with other staff members, or limited to a specific role for each staff member.

Private Duty Nursing

A wholly independent nursing service is given by the private duty nurse, who works directly for a patient. Nursing care may be given in an institution, at the patient's home, or at another place requested by the patient. The patient is the nurse's employer and pays the nurse directly. The nurse is responsible for handling taxes, licenses, and other financial matters relating to self-employment.

A private duty nurse in an institution is subject to the institution's policies and direction and is responsible to the physician or other authority in overall charge of a patient's care. In the home setting, although working under the direction of the patient's physician, the nurse must depend on her own judgment and experience to provide care.

Home Health Care Nursing

The principle of home health care is to provide health care services in the patient's home. The growing number of home health care agencies is mostly the result of the increasing population of elderly persons requiring health care.

Home health care delivers a variety of services by a wide range of providers that can include registered nurses, licensed practical/vocational nurses, social workers, home health aides, and physical, occupational, and speech therapists.

Industrial/Occupational Nursing

Factories and manufacturing plants have had limited in-plant nursing services for years. Generally first-aid oriented—with an emphasis on accident prevention—services were established in response to the influence of labor unions. Today, as business and industry provide more services for their employees, nursing opportunities in the industrial sector are increasing. With a concern for good health now a national issue, other industries, white collar as well as blue collar, have installed health-oriented facilities and staffs that address on-the-job accident treatment and prevention, and broader issues as well. Physical exams, screening tests, diagnostic surveys, and health education are common services offered.

Hospice Nursing

The hospice movement is dedicated to making the inevitable death of terminally ill patients dignified and humane. It provides compassionate care and understanding in settings that are comfortable, familiar, and nonthreatening.

Nurses who work with dying patients require a very special understanding of themselves and of their patient's unique place in a world that has become difficult for the patient to accept and understand. The nurse in a hospice setting must also be able to interact with the patient's family while not interfering with the patient's and family's personal relationships and business.

Hospice care is based on a philosophy that can be implemented in a variety of settings. Most often hospice services are provided in the home; however it can also be found in hospitals, long-term care facilities, and other health care settings.

School Nursing

School nursing, like nursing services offered by business and industry, has expanded from the delivery of simple first aid, immunizations, and health screenings to a comprehensive program of prevention, treatment, and education. Depending on the size of the school district, a school nursing department can be small or extensive. A single nurse may serve a number of schools, or each school may have its own nurse. The registered nurse in a school or schools functions independently and is generally under the authority of a physician appointed by the school district's board of education. LP/VNs assist the registered nurse with routine screening programs and daily activities associated with school nursing.

Nursing Homes

The rise in population of elderly Americans has accounted for a significant increase in the need for nursing and convalescent homes to care for older people who are unable to provide for themselves at home but who do not require hospitalization. The need for nurses to staff these institutions has risen accordingly.

A nursing home may be privately endowed or funded by local or state money. It may be for profit or not for profit, but it must be licensed by the state in which it is located. The services provided may range from simple custodial caretaking to complete medical and rehabilitative care. In general, nursing care is supervised by a registered nurse who is responsible for the overall care of clients under the direction of a physician on call. LP/VNs are often employed as charge nurses and direct the day-to-day delivery of nursing care.

Veterans Administration and Armed Forces Nursing

The Veterans Administration's hospital system is the nation's largest, and its hospitals are some of the biggest. They are federally operated hospitals that care for veterans of the U.S. armed forces. Many of them are affiliated with schools of medicine and nursing.

A wide range of job experience, potential for travel, and other benefits are associated with employment in Veterans Administration hospitals.

The United States Army offers career opportunities to licensed practical nurses in the Army Medical Corp. Applicants must be U.S. citizens, 17 to 34 years old, and graduates of 1-year practical/vocational nursing programs who hold current licenses.

The navy, army, and air force have career nursing opportunities for registered nurses (RN).

Whether you choose to work in a hospital or any one of the many other types of health care facilities, employers have certain general expectations of their employees. Knowing what employers expect of employees in any work situation will help you understand and accept your new role.

Employer Expectations

Employers expect you to have a theoretical basis for what you do so that you can understand the care you give, how to give it, what is expected from it, and what the effects of that care are, so that, if necessary, additional action can be taken.

Your employer will expect you to contribute to patient care by participating in conferences, serving on committees, and maintaining the skills required of the position.

Your employer will expect you to know how to keep records of your activities. Because charts are so important to patient care and as legal documents, skills in charting procedures are definitely expected. Although most employers allow time to learn their specific system, once the system is learned, you will be expected to keep accurate, legible, and technically and grammatically correct records.

Your nursing skills and how well you perform them will be expected to be comparable with other nurses who have the same level of education and experience. An employer will expect you to complete your assignments within a reasonable period of time.

Employers expect a nurse who cannot perform a skill, or who needs help, to ask for assistance. Employers will expect you to function within the law and according to the job description for your position.

Employers expect you to assume responsibility for your work. This includes specific obligations spelled out in the hiring agreement and other implied obligations such as honesty, promptness, and commitment to the job.

Employers expect you to support their philosophy and implement the objectives of the organization. They expect you to be loyal to the organization and fair in your relationships with them.

As you begin your career in practical/vocational nursing, your skills and abilities may not yet match all of your employer's expectations. Making the transition from being a student to being a productive employee who is able to meet an employer's expectations can be a difficult process.

If you decide to become an employee in the institution where you were assigned for clinical experience, the transition may be relatively easy; if you decide to accept a position in an institution that is unfamiliar to you, the transition may be more difficult. In either case, there are some transitional challenges that will confront you as a beginning nurse. Being prepared to meet these challenges will help you adjust to your first job as an LPN or an LVN.

Transitional Challenges

There are many differences between being a student nurse and being a graduate LP/VN. As a student, the conditions under which you are learning are controlled to provide the maximum educational benefit to you and your classmates. Your clinical assignments are selected to contribute to your educational development. Your clinical instructor is legally responsible for your performance in the clinical area and is there to help you resolve problems and answer questions. As a graduate, your assignments will be based on the needs of the patients and the needs of your employer. You will be responsible and accountable for your own actions. And you will be expected to carry out your assignments within the allotted time.

Making these adjustments from student to employee may be difficult. You will not always have the same amount of time you had as a student to spend with patients. Your work load and the pace at which you will be expected to carry out your assignments will be increased. Some experienced members of the nursing team may help you during his transition period; others may not.

Expect to have some mixed feelings—some very positive and others less so. You will be excited to finally have the chance to put what you have learned to actual use, but you might also be a bit nervous about it. You may feel that there is more work than you can handle. You may have difficulty adjusting to the leadership and management style of your supervisor. But remember, you successfully made similar adjustments when you began your nursing program, and you can do so again.

Some of the techniques that help ease the transition from student to employee include being honest about your limitations but not shirking your share of the work. If you find that you are getting behind schedule, let your supervisor know. You may want to ask an experienced nursing team member for suggestions on how to better organize your work. Observe how experienced nurses organize their schedules so that assignments are completed on time. You might ask your supervisor to evaluate your performance on a daily or weekly basis and use that information to improve your practice. Take every opportunity you can to learn more about your patient's medical conditions and their nursing needs. Admit your mistakes and learn from them. Be prepared to put in the extra time needed to complete your assignments without expecting to be paid for that time. In a surprisingly short time, you will make the adjustment and feel the satisfaction that comes from being accepted as a contributing member of the nursing team.

Self-assessment

Now that you have reviewed some of the career opportunities in nursing, employer expectations, and transitional challenges, you should assess your self. Self-esteem and sound skills lend encouragement and confidence to one's outlook and tasks, whereas lack of self-esteem and poor skills can undermine one's confidence. The ability to make an objective analysis of yourself will help to point up areas of strength and areas where improvement may be needed. The key is to see yourself as best you can without the influence of your own beliefs or wishes about how you think you are or would like to be. An accurate self-assessment is not always easy, but the rewards make the effort worthwhile.

A review of your clinical strengths and weaknesses is an important consideration when you are thinking about the type of nursing you would prefer to do. If you seem to have a special ability to work with older people, you may consider employment in a long-term care facility. If you enjoyed your clinical experiences on the surgical unit in a general hospital, that may be the best place for you to begin your career.

You should assess your personal health and physical condition. If you have a health problem or physical condition that limits your activities, you should avoid seeking a position that would adversely affect your own health.

You should assess your work habits, how you prefer to dress, and other personal characteristics. Working in a situation that requires you to behave very differently from the way you usually behave can cause a great deal of stress and personal conflict.

Finally, you should assess your personal and interpersonal characteristics. On p. 220 is a list of some characteristics to look for. As you read them, ask yourself how the item applies to you—Always, Usually, Never—and mark the appropriate space next to the item. On completion, review the list with someone who knows you well, and ask what the answer should be. Compare the responses. The results are not scientific but they will give you an indication of your self perception and how others may see you. Use them to alter those aspects of yourself that may need changing. Evaluations from instructors during the course of your program can also be used to help judge yourself.

Finding a Position

The job-seeking process should be started in the months preceding your graduation.

Personal and Interpersonal Characteristics Assessment

Personal Characteristics	Always	Usually	Never
1. I accept responsibility for my work	____	____	____
2. I welcome criticism	____	____	____
3. I tell the truth	____	____	____
4. I don't waste time	____	____	____
5. I am patient with myself	____	____	____
6. I like solving problems	____	____	____
7. I am organized	____	____	____
8. I know my own limits	____	____	____
9. I am comfortable with rules and regulations	____	____	____
10. I accept change	____	____	____
11. I do not have to be told what to do	____	____	____
12. I do more than I'm asked	____	____	____
13. I control my emotions	____	____	____
14. I have a good sense of humor	____	____	____
15. I ask for help when I need it	____	____	____

Interpersonal Characteristics	Always	Usually	Never
1. I enjoy working with others	____	____	____
2. I am a good listener	____	____	____
3. I don't mind sharing credit with others	____	____	____
4. I am patient with others	____	____	____
5. I keep promises	____	____	____
6. I like meeting strangers	____	____	____
7. I like being in charge	____	____	____
8. I like talking about work with colleagues	____	____	____
9. I am tolerant of others' mistakes	____	____	____
10. I treat everyone as an individual	____	____	____
11. I go out of my way to help co-workers	____	____	____
12. I like being a part of a group	____	____	____
13. I keep judgments of others to myself	____	____	____

Your first task should be to develop a list of names and places where you might expect to find employment opportunities when you complete your program. This list should consist of the names of people and institutions you've met or learned about while in your program. As your graduation approaches, check with those on the list from time to time. Ask about the present hiring situation, whether it has changed from the last time you inquired, and what the future looks like. Begin to cultivate relationships with people who are employed at the health care facilities where you believe you'd like to work.

According to some statistics, as many as 80 percent of all jobs are obtained through personal contacts. Networking—the deliberate effort to make connections among people for a variety of interests, including employment opportunities—is a popular method of making personal contacts. Networking may be casual, as when a group of health care workers meet from time to time over coffee to talk, or it may be more formal, as when groups meet with the specific intention of exchanging information. Look for networking opportunities in your program, among graduates, and others in the health care field in your community.

You'll also learn about employment opportunities by talking with and listening to fellow students, your instructors, and others associated with your program. When you hear something that sounds interesting, make a note to yourself to follow it up with an inquiry.

If your program has a placement service, it can be an invaluable resource. Use it to get information about your local employment market before you're ready to begin applying for a job. Stay in touch with employment developments in your area through the placement service. When the time comes to begin making serious inquiries and applications, you will be up to date.

Most schools have a "Job Opportunities" bulletin board, where notices about employment are posted. Make the board a regular stop and watch for new offers to appear.

Begin reading the classified section of your local newspaper. Major papers may have a special section for health care. You'll get a good idea of the hiring trends by the number of ads that appear. Even when ads don't apply directly to you, they can be a good source of names of local institutions and private practitioners to add to your contact list.

Most communities have employment agencies, and larger cities have placement agencies that specialize in health care personnel. Either kind of agency is a good resource, but those which specialize are likely to have more listings and better contacts with employers because of their specialization. If you register with an agency, your name will be available when applicants are needed to fill newly opened positions. Commercial employment agencies charge for their services, usually a percentage of the first year's salary. In some cases the employer may pay this charge; in others, it is paid by the employee, that is, you. Ask what the fee is and who will pay it before signing an agreement with an employment agency.

Evaluating Positions

With many employment opportunities now available to licensed practical/ vocational nurses, considering a position includes knowing as much about it as possible before making a decision.

Each facet of every opening you are considering should be examined separately. You should not make any presumptions about any aspect of a job you are thinking of applying for, regardless of what outside appearances may suggest. It does not follow, for example, that a beautiful prestigious hospital pays the highest salaries, although, of course, it might.

Investigate each employment opportunity on its own merits, paying close attention to all its parts. They include the job description, salary, benefits, work hours, and many other matters that will directly influence your working life and often your whole life. For example, poor working conditions can make one unhappy, and unhappiness does not stay at your place of employment when you go home.

Specific items to consider when evaluating employment opportunities include the following. You may wish to add items of personal concern to the list.

Wages

Your earning power is determined by your credentials on the one hand and by what the job market offers in the form of salary on the other. Ideally, you should earn the maximum salary or wages possible for your level of education and experience, with the salary or wages increasing with your experience. But pay rates vary for a number of reasons.

Generally, regional salaries and wages will be similar because employers are competing for the same prospective employees. Where rates vary, other inducements may be offered to make up the difference. Frequently the inducements—benefits—are as important or even more so than the salary or wages alone.

Be cautious when you see above-average salaries or wages for a position you believe you are qualified for. There is usually a good reason for salaries or wages to be noticeably above a regional average. The job description for the position may call for responsibilities and competencies that are beyond your qualifications. Or the wages may be offered because of a high staff turnover that is the result of difficult working conditions. In the cost-conscious health care field, money that does not have to be spent, seldom is.

Carefully study the salary ranges in your area and learn why those which vary do so. Find out what the maximum starting salaries are, what the maximum salary that can be earned from each employer is, how long it takes to reach the maximum salary, and what conditions you have to satisfy to qualify for the maximum earnings.

Also, find out what a prospective employer's wage increase policies are. Some may give automatic raises, others may give merit raises, and still others may not give raises at all. Learn how long it takes to qualify for an increase and what is needed to qualify, such as additional education, length of service, or other requirements.

Hours and Shifts

Your intention to work full time or part time, as well as your willingness or ability to work different shifts, will have a great bearing on which employment opportunities to consider. Although certain sections of the country have nursing shortages, and employers in those regions are therefore likely to be more flexible, the general rule is that employers set the conditions to maintain continuity of services. You may find some flexibility even in those instances, however.

Work schedules are devised in a variety of ways, but usually they're based on shifts—generally three 8-hour shifts per day. Many employers either require or offer rotating shifts. The work schedule is also often rotated so that all employees have the opportunity to have some weekends and some holidays off.

Your personal circumstances will dictate which schedules you can work. Be certain before applying for a position that you will be available for the hours and shifts being offered or required.

Employer Reputation

Your evaluation of potential employers should include their reputation for upholding high standards. Good and bad reputations are earned for a reason. Learn your prospective employer's reputation and how it was acquired. Don't accept hearsay. Someone may praise or belittle an institution for totally unjustifiable reasons. Find out for yourself. Ask the opinions of those who have worked or received care there. Ask health care associations and societies about their members. And also ask the employer. Those with good reputations will provide verifiable references, whereas those who have something to hide won't provide such references.

Opportunities for Advancement

Although it may be early in your career to think of advancing beyond the immediate goal of earning your license as a practical/vocational nurse, there may come a time in the future when you'd like to continue your education in nursing. Leave this option open by looking at employment opportunities with employers who offer or encourage employee advancement.

Benefits

Benefits include a wide range of items. Some benefits, such as vacation time, may be considered basic, whereas others, such as day care facilities for employee's children, may be less standard. Look closely at the benefits package of each employer you are considering. Benefits can be a decisive factor in choosing a position. A high salary without certain benefits may result in a lower overall income for you, whereas a lower salary or wage with good benefits may net you more.

Some benefits to look for are insurance (life, health, vision, dental) plans; overtime pay; pension plans; reimbursement for tuition; employee credit union; in-service educational programs; meals; laundry and uniform provision; and vacation, leave of absence, and holiday policies.

Some questions to investigate include the following:

Vacation, Sick Leave, Holidays, and Leave of Absence

- How much time for each of the above is provided?
- Does the time provided increase with length of employment?
- Is the time with or without pay?
- How many and which holidays are included?
- How is a leave of absence granted?
- Is job status affected by a leave of absence?
- How does a leave affect seniority?
- Is maternity leave granted?

Insurance, Credit, and Pension

- Are insurance, credit, and pension plans group or individual plans?
- How soon after employment begins are the plans effective?
- What does each plan offer?
- Who is eligible?
- What are the conditions of eligibility?

- Who pays insurance premiums? How much (full or percentage)?
- Are payments automatic (payroll deducted) or voluntary?
- Is interest charged for credit union loans? How much?
- Is interest paid to credit union members? How much?

Work Environment

- Is the facility convenient to public or private transportation?
- Is safe parking provided? Is it free or pay?
- Are uniforms required? If so, what kind and who provides them?
- Is the facility clean and safe?
- Is equipment and care delivery up to date?
- Do present employees exhibit good morale?

Miscellaneous

- What are the work hours, shifts, and rotation schedules?
- Are meals provided, either free or at employee discounts?
- Is there a cafeteria? What are its condition, service, and fare?
- Is laundry service for uniforms provided or available?
- Does the facility have an orientation program or in-service education program? Does it offer advanced educational opportunities at outside institutions?
- Who pays tuition and costs for advanced education programs?

The Application Process

On graduation, you will have to apply for a job. You can do this informally, by personally visiting prospective places of employment, or more formally—and preferably—by submitting a letter of application with an accompanying resume. The letter assures you that the prospective employer has a written record of your interest, and the resume provides the prospective employer with an outline of your qualifications.

Large institutions with many employees often have personnel departments where it is appropriate to "walk in" to make an application. Also, some employers who advertise may invite walk-ins.

The Letter of Application

A letter of application should be simple and direct. Its objective is to introduce you, announce your interest in employment (naming the position being applied for), briefly state your qualifications, and express your availability. It should be typewritten on one page in standard business letter

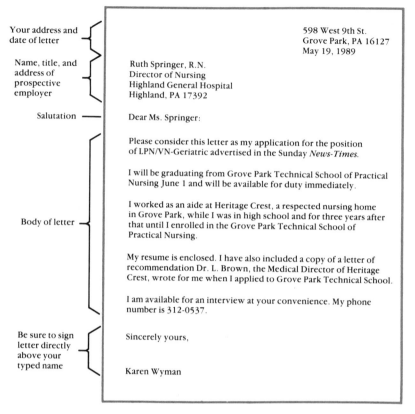

Your address and
date of letter

598 West 9th St.
Grove Park, PA 16127
May 19, 1989

Name, title, and
address of
prospective
employer

Ruth Springer, R.N.
Director of Nursing
Highland General Hospital
Highland, PA 17392

Salutation

Dear Ms. Springer:

Body of letter

Please consider this letter as my application for the position
of LPN/VN-Geriatric advertised in the Sunday *News-Times.*

I will be graduating from Grove Park Technical School of Practical
Nursing June 1 and will be available for duty immediately.

I worked as an aide at Heritage Crest, a respected nursing home
in Grove Park, while I was in high school and for three years after
that until I enrolled in the Grove Park Technical School of
Practical Nursing.

My resume is enclosed. I have also included a copy of a letter of
recommendation Dr. L. Brown, the Medical Director of Heritage
Crest, wrote for me when I applied to Grove Park Technical School.

I am available for an interview at your convenience. My phone
number is 312-0537.

Be sure to sign
letter directly
above your
typed name

Sincerely yours,

Karen Wyman

Figure 12-1. Sample application letter.

form. It should be free of grammatical and spelling errors. Figure 12-1 is an
example of an application letter.

The Resume

Like your letter of application, your resume represents you to your prospective employer. Neatness, clarity, legibility, and organization on paper reflect similar personal qualities. Although you may wish to write your own resume, the general availability of resume writing services makes the task much simpler.

If you don't have access to a resume writing service, you might want to consider engaging a secretary or other person with the skills to produce one for you, rather than trusting your own typing and organization.

Whether you write your own resume or have someone write it for you,

Sandra Melanie Lewis, L.P.N.
1038 University Avenue
Boulder, Colorado 80302
303-264-0537

Immediate Goal:
Employment as a licensed practical nurse in the geriatric section
of a major area hospital

Career Goal:
To provide quality nursing care for older adults in long-term
care

Education:
1989: Arapahoe Hospital, Boulder, Colorado; L.P.N.
1987: Boulder High School, Boulder, Colorado; H.S. diploma

Licenses:
Licensed Practical Nurse, State of Colorado, 1989

Experience:
1984-87: Nurses aide (parttime), Boulder Nursing Home, Boulder,
Colorado; elderly long-term care facility; assisted LPNs after
school and weekends

1987-88; Aide (fulltime), Boulder Nursing Home, Boulder, Colorado

Memberships and Honors:
HOSA Club; Boulder County 4-H Club, Secretary, 1985-87; Scholarship,
Hopkins Pharmaceutical Company, 1987 (awarded to Outstanding
Student in Health Occupations Students of America)

Availability: Immediate

References:
Available on request

Figure 12-2. Sample resume.

it should follow a standardized format. If you're doing your own, get the information you need from the reference section of your library or from the placement office at your school. Don't simply write a "homemade" resume; it will stand out, but not in the way a good resume is intended to. See Figure 12-2 for an example of a solid resume.

The following categories of information should be included on your resume:

- Name, address, and telephone number
- Immediate goal
- Career goal
- Education
- Licenses
- Experience (work and volunteer)
- Memberships and honors
- Reference availability

The Interview

The decision to hire a candidate for a job is made within the first 30 seconds of the first meeting between the candidate and the person doing the hiring, according to one report. Whether this finding is completely accurate or not, it underscores the fact that when you go for a job interview, you should assume that your appearance and how you present yourself will make an important impression on the interviewer.

If you've done your "homework" and have taken the time to learn as much as you can about the employer you're seeing, you'll have a good idea of what the interviewer is looking for in an applicant and how you can prepare yourself to meet those expectations. In general, a few simple guidelines will be sufficient:

- Dress appropriately. You are applying for a job. This means that what you wear should be "businesslike." You should present a serious, capable image that is neither frivolous nor too casual.
- Be well groomed. Combed hair, clean skin, and an overall appearance that shows you take good care of yourself will also signal to an employer what kind of care you are likely to give patients.
- Be pleasant and polite but avoid forcing an unnatural "charm." Act yourself, not someone you aren't.
- Show interest in the employer and the job. It will be helpful if you demonstrate a knowledge of the employer and the employer's needs.
- Don't be too concerned about nervousness. Most interviewers expect this, particularly in new entrants to the job market.
- Remember that at the same time the interviewer is listening to your answers to questions, he is observing how you respond and is also judging how well you interact with people.

You will show your interest in the employer if you ask questions, but be sure to ask them at appropriate times. Although it is acceptable to inquire about the wages and benefits the job offers, for example, it is not appropriate to ask about them before the subjects come up. Normally this would be well into the interview. The early part of the interview should focus on the employer, the position offered, its requirements, and your own qualifications for the job.

You will be given the opportunity to ask questions. Prepare a list of good questions ahead of time to avoid the possibility of "going blank," which could be interpreted as disinterest. When given the opportunity to ask questions, you can ask about issues such as salary, vacations, and other matters that apply directly to you, if they have not already been addressed.

The Job Offer

When all of your employment investigation has been done, the letters of application written, the resumes sent, and the interviews completed, one or more of the prospective employers you applied to will offer you a job.

Review each offer before accepting or rejecting it to make sure the choice you make is the one you want. If you've already made up your mind that you will accept, do so. If you're uncertain, tell the employer that you will make your decision by a specific date or time. At this point in your career, at the very outset of your practice, you must be as sure as possible that your choice of an employer is what you want. It is far better for you to take the time at the beginning to assure yourself that the job being offered is for you than to find out after you're hired that it's not, and then have to face resigning and beginning anew. As a graduate practical/vocational nurse in a field that needs you, you don't have to take the first opportunity that comes along if it's not what you want. However, avoid "closing the door" to a first job on the basis of unrealistic demands. Although the perfect job may be waiting for you, it's more likely you will have to make some compromises.

On the Job

Once you are hired, a new round of learning begins. You'll be learning your employer's routine, your specific duties, the names and faces of co-workers and patients, and scores of other details. Your confidence in yourself and your competence will get you through the rough parts, and understanding from those you're working with will help to smooth the transition. You can expect some highs and lows, but you should always know that in a surprisingly short time, the insecurity of being new will be replaced by poise and self-assurance.

But confidence in yourself alone will not guarantee satisfactory performance. Your own standards should be high, perhaps even higher than those your employer sets, so that your work will never come into question and your ability will never fall short of what's expected.

Accept the responsibilities you are given. Do your work to the best of your ability, with interest and commitment. Be punctual and reliable, and if illness or interruption prevents you from reporting to work, notify your employer as soon as possible. Show a willingness to learn by asking questions when you are uncertain, and be equally willing to share when someone comes to you for help. Abide by the regulations set by your employer, and if you have serious differences with them, seek to correct the situation through proper channels; don't snipe, gossip, or bad-mouth about something that upsets you—do something about it, but in the appropriate manner. You are not only working *for* your employer; you are also working *with* him to provide the service that is the basis for the economic security of both of you.

On the job, you have two roles: yourself as you and yourself as nurse-employee. Your nurse-employee role must come first. When you go to work, leave your personal problems behind. But positive personal characteristics such as honesty, courtesy, good humor, compassion, and understanding are valuable assets as an individual and as a nurse, and you should exhibit them at work, just as you would elsewhere.

Politeness in person or on the phone, in greeting people who are new to you or in your relationships with those you see regularly, is also important. Showing good manners on any occasion, whether in an employee cafeteria or in a patient's room, helps to set an example and a tone that inspires similar behavior from others.

Avoiding gossip about your institution, its staff, or your patients is more than desirable; it is essential. Backbiting, grousing, complaining, and speaking ill of anyone or anything not only poisons others' attitudes but darkens your own point of view. Use caution when talking about personal work issues. Others may not share your views, and it is not fair to impose yours if they are negative.

You will always be working directly or indirectly with others. How closely you work together will vary. Some will have authority over you; others will be under your supervision. Some you may rarely see, whereas others may be at your side constantly. Good relationships with others will depend heavily on what you do to keep them good. In general, what you put into a relationship is what you get out of it.

There may be times when you witness care or are asked to deliver care that is below the standards of good nursing or health care. Your first obligation is to your patients. If the care you see is truly substandard and can be verified, you should act to prevent it. Report the situation to your supervisor.

Don't act on your own to correct the situation, because the possibility exists that you're not seeing all the factors involved. Health care at any level always includes the potential of serious consequences, the worst being the possible consequence of death.

Dealing with people will be the major part of your work. However, in the process of providing care, you will also be responsible for such things as dressings, medications, instruments, machines, and a long list of supplies. They belong to your employer and are expressly for use in the delivery of services to the patients being cared for. Their misuse or misappropriation for a staff member's private use, without permission, is unethical and illegal.

To avoid problems over the use of equipment and supplies, abide by your employer's regulations regarding them. Fill out the forms that may be required. Make accurate counts when taking inventories or requisitioning supplies. Return unused items to their proper place. File breakage or failed equipment reports. In short, do everything you are supposed to do regarding the use of facilities and supplies.

Health care facilities of every size are continuously battling increasing costs. Any loss, no matter how insignificant it may seem—making an unauthorized long-distance phone call, taking a set of linens or a towel, or using medications for personal use, for example—raises costs. When an employer's costs are excessive, cost-cutting procedures—including staff cuts—may become necessary. Your job will depend on your employer's ability to pay you. How you use your employer's facilities, equipment, and supplies will affect that ability.

With your career aspirations in mind, take advantage of opportunities to advance. If you need additional classes, in-service training, or experience, accept the added effort, knowing that no advancement is possible without it.

Resignation

There may come a time when you decide to leave your position. This decision should never be made without careful study. A brief upset or disagreement with someone is certainly not grounds for leaving, although a long period of inability to get along in an institution or with staff members may suggest a change for the better. If you decide to resign, always do so in the manner set forth by your employer. If no prescribed form is established, write a letter of resignation. Give ample notice—2 weeks is standard—so that your employer can find a replacement for you. No matter what the circumstances of your departure, don't infuse the situation with ill will. You will be looking for another job, if not immediately, then at some time in the future. Your employer's recommendation will be invaluable.

A letter of resignation should be simple and direct, stating the fact that

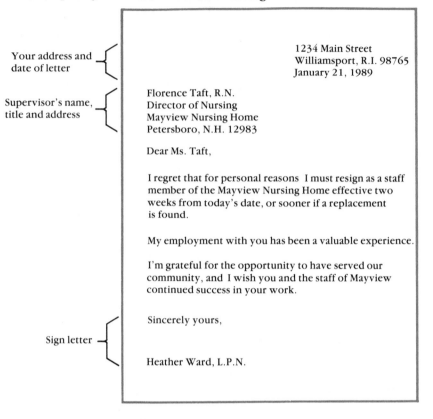

Your address and
date of letter

1234 Main Street
Williamsport, R.I. 98765
January 21, 1989

Supervisor's name,
title and address

Florence Taft, R.N.
Director of Nursing
Mayview Nursing Home
Petersboro, N.H. 12983

Dear Ms. Taft,

I regret that for personal reasons I must resign as a staff
member of the Mayview Nursing Home effective two
weeks from today's date, or sooner if a replacement
is found.

My employment with you has been a valuable experience.

I'm grateful for the opportunity to have served our
community, and I wish you and the staff of Mayview
continued success in your work.

Sincerely yours,

Sign letter

Heather Ward, L.P.N.

Figure 12-3.   Sample resignation letter.

you are resigning, the effective date, giving the reasons (elaborate details
are unnecessary), and closing on a positive note. A sample is shown in
Figure 12-3.

Dismissal

Dismissal from a position is a possibility that is not always based on
employer-employee incompatibility. There are economic and other reasons
for cutting staffs, and you have no control over them. If you "fall under the
axe" of budget cuts or other administrative changes, such as consolidation
of departments, you must accept them. Often an employer who adjusts staff
will have alternative jobs within the institution or, if not, will try to help
employees find new positions, but employers are under no obligation.

On the other hand, a dismissal for cause, based on dishonesty, improper performance of duty, insubordination, illegal acts, excessive lateness or absences, or other substantiated causes, is something every nurse can do something about before it happens. Adherence to high standards is the best defense against charges of any kind.

If a dismissal is warranted, even though it might be disputed by the employee, the employer has certain options, depending on the nature of the cause for dismissal. The options will vary from employer to employer. A serious charge such as theft can result in an immediate dismissal with forfeiture of all benefits. A less serious matter, such as constantly arriving late for work, although grounds for dismissal if not corrected, is not likely to result in such drastic measures. In most cases, the dismissed employee may have the right to appeal.

Your Budget

Budgeting your income is largely a personal matter. You may already have a system for managing your money. If not, seek help for your specific needs from someone who understands the process. A budget does not have to be complex, but it should cover all areas of your income and expenses, the two major divisions of any budget.

If your position as an LP/VN is your first major employment, be sure to make the distinction between personal and professional (or business) expenses in your budget. Also, since you may be paying local, state, or federal taxes for the first time, get advice from an expert regarding what records you have to keep, how much you must pay, and how the taxes are to be paid. Private duty nurses are responsible for paying their own taxes and for getting licenses required for private duty practice.

Other money matters for you to consider include savings or investment programs, personal insurance (life; health; liability), and the establishment of a good credit rating.

Guidance in these matters is recommended, even if you must consult a professional.

Career Advancement

As your practical nurse program draws to an end, you should feel secure that your career as a nurse is well on its way. Now is a good time to think further in terms of what the future might hold. Goals are incentives to self-fulfillment and to a better, more comfortable life.

Earning your license and a position as an LP/VN may be the goals you have always wanted, and now, as the time you'll reach them comes close, they alone may be totally satisfying to you. However, this accomplishment is proof of what you are capable of achieving. Your success may lead you to strive even higher. If so, numerous opportunities are available.

Higher goals do not necessarily mean the need to earn higher degrees. As you gain experience as a practical/vocational nurse, keep an eye on your future by reading professional nursing journals such as the *Journal of Practical Nursing* and *Nursing*. Stay abreast of developments that affect your work and the health care field in general. Attend in-service education programs whenever they are offered, keeping a record of them and updating your credentials.

Various organizations sponsor conventions and workshops. They may be offered locally or in another city. Attend them whenever possible, even if you must do so on your own time. If you show your determination to keep pace with nursing and a willingnes to go out of your way to do so, you may get cooperation and time off from your employer. The least you will get will be your employer's respect for your enthusiasm and interest.

Continuing education units (CEUs) (one CEU equals 10 hours of qualified instruction in an approved program) are sometimes given by continuing education programs. Earned CEUs are an indiciation to your employer and others of your career commitment. CEUs are also required for license renewal in some states.

Refresher courses are also a means to maintain and improve skills and knowledge. They may be offered by your own program and by your employer. Treat them as opportunities to advance.

After you've been employed for a time, you may be offered the opportunity to specialize in a specific health care area. If you think that your theoretical knowledge has not kept up with the practical experience you've gained on the job, and if in-service training, refresher courses, and reading fail to get you to the competency you want, additional study may be the answer. Consider enrolling in an accredited course offered by a college or university. "Accredited" means that a course or program has been reviewed by an organization or accrediting body and has been found to meet the standards set by that body. Accrediting standards generally mean that standards are above minimum standards as set, for example, by a state licensing authority.

A simple and painless way to maintain an educational program is to take extension courses offered on television, usually on public service channels. Before committing yourself, make certain that you will receive credit for the course.

Finally, you may wish to make a major advance in your nursing career by becoming a registered nurse. Registered nurse (RN) programs vary in length and complexity. A full 4-year course of study at a college or university will lead to a bachelor of science in nursing (BSN) degree and the qualification to take the RN licensing exam.

An associate degree in nursing (ADN) is usually earned at a college, university, or junior or community college. It is a 2-year degree that qualifies the student to take the RN licensing exam in most states.

Diploma programs are sponsored by hospitals or other institutions and lead to diplomas from the sponsoring institution and the qualification to take the RN exam.

Collective Bargaining

Certain issues regarding your employment will be out of your direct control but within your indirect control. They are the conditions affecting your job such as wage scales, work hours, working conditions, and other matters that are of daily concern. Nurses' unions are organizations which, by representing nurses and bargaining with employers, reach agreements that ideally are in everyone's best interest. The process is called collective bargaining.

If you join a union, and if that union is acknowledged as the bargaining representative at your place of employment, your wishes will be conveyed to management (your employer) through the activities of the union. But you must first belong to the union and then be active in it for the process to be effective.

Unions work for the benefit of their members. Any issue can be advanced by a union, but in general unions are involved in wage and hour matters, health and safety issues, discrimination issues of all kinds, and the formulation of contracts between employers and union members that incorporate these items.

Joining a union is a personal choice. Whether or not you accept an offer to join is up to you. Before deciding either to join or not to join, look closely into what your decision would mean to you, your employment, and your career.

Grievances

No occupation or job is without its grievances (problems). It's not a good idea to look for them, especially at the beginning of your career, when your attention should be on learning and performance, but you should be aware that they may appear from time to time. They may cover a range of serious matters, such as health and safety or discrimination on the basis of sex, race, religion or other factor. There may be less serious issues of only passing concern. Some can be solved on the spot; others may require a lengthy process to settle.

Most employers will have some form of grievance procedure (prob- lem-settling process) for you to follow to rectify problems. In some institu- tions the process may be a part of a contract worked out by the union representing the workers there. At other establishments it may be as simple as calling the problem to the attention of a supervisor.

Learn the process that is used at your institution or place of employ- ment, because without it, small, even petty problems could grow out of proportion, and already large problems could become serious. Complaining about a problem accomplishes nothing if it's not done through the proper channels, whereas a legitimate complaint that reaches an authority who can do something about it gets action.

Burnout

The term "burnout" describes a condition characterized by a sense of hope- lessness about one's job that is brought about by chronic stress. It decreases performance on the job and carries over into one's personal life. It can be the result of highly stressful working conditions or stressful relationships among staff.

Physical and psychological symptoms accompany burnout. Physical symptoms may include exhaustion, fatigue, headaches, susceptibility to colds, and the inability to sleep. Psychological symptoms may include quick loss of temper, decreased ability to make decisions, guilt, anger, and depression.

At least part of the stress that produces burnout comes from the inability of those who suffer it to match what they expect of themselves to what time and conditions let them deliver. Candidates for burnout include the nurse who wants to provide ideal nursing care but is prevented from doing so because there isn't enough time for each patient and the nurse whose aim is to promote health but is faced every day with dying patients.

Often the nurse who has reached this point solves the problem by quitting nursing. This is a dramatic and unnecessary solution.

The issue of burnout is a growing concern in health care. As a new member of the health care team, you can do something now to manage the stress that may lie ahead by being prepared. Discuss problems openly with co-workers and supervisors. Learn to share your feelings and listen to others in return. If the area of health care you are about to enter is one of known high stress, find out from the beginning what those who are already in it do to manage theirs. Don't shoulder a burden that is not yours to carry alone.

Discussion Questions/Learning Activities

1. In addition to nursing opportunities listed in this chapter, list other places where LP/VNs may work in your community. (Your local newspaper may help you with this question.)
2. What is the salary range for the LP/VNs in various health care facilities in your community? (Your local newspaper and health facility personnel offices can help you answer this question.) Prepare your resume for a prospective employer.
3. Ask a classmate to conduct a mock interview with you. Analyze
4. your ability to ask clear, concise, and relevant questions. Ask your interviewer to give you their impressions of how well you presented yourself during the mock interview. well you presented yourself during the mock interview.
5. Think about how you will dress for an interview. Your librarian can direct you to reference books that discuss dressing for an interview.
6. Ask one or two experienced nurses about their transition from student to employee. What did they find most difficult? What would they recommend to make this transition less difficult?
7. List several things that you can do now to prepare to make the transition from student to employee.
8. Review the stress management techniques in Appendix C. How could you use some of these techniques to help you avoid "burnout"?
9. Prepare a list of the pros and cons of union membership. Compare your list with those of your classmates.
10 Describe your nursing career goals. What position and responsibility do you want in 1 year, in 5 years, and in 10 years? What will you have to do to achieve these goals? Are these goals realistic? Do you have the ability to achieve them? What changes (personal, educational, social) might you have to make to achieve your goals?

References

American Nurses' Association. The Grievance Procedure. Kansas City, MO, The Association, 1985.

Anastas L: Your Career in Nursing. New York, National League for Nursing, 1984.

Benner P: From Novice to Expert: Excellence and Power in Clinical Nursing Practice. Menlo Park, CA, Addison-Wesley, 1984.

Grippando GM: Nursing Perspective and Issues. Albany, NY, Delmar, 1986.

Hamilton JM, Kiefer ME: Survival Skills for the New Nurse. Philadelphia, JB Lippincott, 1986.

Hanger TI: Designing Your Nursing Career: Finding a Terrific First Job. Los Altos, CA, National Nursing Review, 1986.

Health Care Education Associates Staff. Writing the Nursing Resume. St. Louis, CV Mosby, 1986.

Smythe EEM: Surviving Nursing. Menlo Park, CA, Addison-Wesley, 1984.

13 Current Issues and Future Concerns

Objectives

When you complete this chapter, you should be able to:

Discuss several methods through which you can maintain your competence in nursing practice.

Critically analyze an announcement for a continuing education program.

Identify the advantages and disadvantages of mandatory continuing education for nurse license renewal.

Define institutional licensure and describe the reasons supporting or rejecting this type of license.

Prepare a list of activities you can do that may contribute to alleviate the nursing shortage.

Debate the right of nurses to go on strike.

List and describe some of the major issues and future concerns of nurses and nursing.

Define the term "entry into practice" and discuss the current controversy.

Take and defend your position on current issues in nursing.

It is impossible in one chapter to present or thoroughly discuss all the current issues and future concerns that face you as you begin your career in practical/vocational nursing. Because nursing, medicine, and health care are dynamic, the principles and philosophies that guide them and the technology used to apply them are being adapted continuously to social, cultural, and scientific changes.

What you know today will get you started, but you will have to continually strive to adapt to social, cultural, and scientific changes. You must actively participate in resolving issues and concerns that will affect your career as a licensed practical/vocational nurse now and in the future.

Maintaining Competence

Several sources predict that what you learn this year will be obsolete in less than 6 years. Your nursing program has prepared you with the minimum competencies needed to enter the practice of practical/vocational nursing, but maintaining your competencies will require attention throughout your entire career.

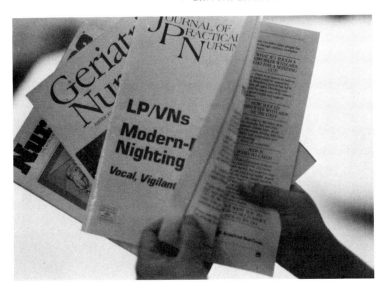

Journals provide current information that can help you keep up with changes in the field of nursing.

Maintaining competence through informal educational experiences is one of the most frequently used methods for keeping up with changes in nursing. Reading journals, attending staff development programs offered by your employer, learning new procedures or techniques from those skilled in their performance, reading patient charts, listening to physicians as they discuss treatment options, and learning to use new and different equipment will help you remain competent in your nursing skills.

Another method for maintaining competence is through formal continuing education. Formal continuing education includes lectures, workshops, seminars, college courses, and independent study programs designed by nursing associations. Sponsors of continuing education programs include hospitals, nursing homes, colleges and universities, and nursing and health care associations.

Sponsors can apply to nursing organizations such as the American Nurses' Association, the National Federation of Licensed Practical Nurses, the National Association for Practical Nurse Education and Service, the National League for Nursing, and the state board of nursing for program approval. Approved programs may offer continuing education units (CEUs). A CEU is the equivalent of 10 contact hours of participation in an approved continuing education program. A contact hour is equal to 50 minutes.

The National Association for Practical Nurse Education and Service (NAPNES) offers several formal continuing education opportunities. NAPNES also provides a Continuing Education Record Keeping System (CERKS) for both members and nonmembers. The system records your continuing education contact hours and supplies transcripts when you want or need to document your participation in continuing education programs. For additional information on continuing education programs or CERKS, you can write to NAPNES. (Refer to Appendix F for the NAPNES address.)

When selecting a continuing education program, you should consider those which apply directly to your learning needs. You will want to determine the purpose of the program, the objectives, the content, the teaching-learning methods, and faculty qualifications. You will also want to know whether the program is approved to offer CEUs and what organization gave that approval.

A current issue that will no doubt become more and more important is the controversy over whether continuing education should be voluntary or mandatory. Those who believe that continuing education should be voluntary assert that continuing education is a responsibility of all nurses and that laws should not dictate how this responsibility is met. Those who favor mandatory continuing education believe that this is the only way to ensure that nurses will keep their knowledge current.

The nurse practice acts of at least 11 states require a specific number of contact hours in continuing education for license renewal as a practical/vocational nurse. Other states do not yet have a mandatory continuing education requirement. This is one of the current issues that will affect your nursing practice and one in which you should become involved. Learn the reasons for both mandatory and voluntary continuing education and the implications of each. When the issue is presented in your state or place of employment, you will be prepared to try to influence decisions that will benefit you, your colleagues, and your future.

Advanced Degrees

At some future point in your career as a practical/vocational nurse, you may decide to continue your education in nursing. Whether you choose a diploma nursing school, an associate degree program, or a program offering a baccalaureate degree in nursing, you should weigh all your options. Often what seems the easiest path is not the best for you. Discuss your career goals with counselors at various schools and with your supervisors. Be certain that the educational program you choose will contribute to achieving your goals.

Many programs that prepare students for the registered nurse licensing examination offer special programs for licensed practical/vocational nurse. Some of these special programs can be completed in a relatively short time, and some are offered on a part-time basis for students who do not have the time or cannot afford full-time study. Explore all the educational opportunities open to you so that when the time comes for you to finally make a decision, you will have all the facts and can select the option that is best for you.

Employer tuition assistance plans and educational grants and loans can assist in financing your advanced degree. Scholarships may also be available. Employer tuition assistance plans and some scholarships may require that you agree to work for a particular institution for a specific period. Be sure you understand the conditions associated with financial assistance and be prepared to fulfill any promise you make.

Earning an advanced degree requires a commitment at least equal to the one that you have made in your practical/vocational nursing program. Make your plans to return to school well in advance of the start of the classes, and organize your personal life and work schedule so that you can be a successful student.

Current Issues in Licensure

At the present time, nurses are licensed to practice nursing by the state board of nursing. Institutional licensure means that a hospital or other health care providers would be granted the authority to regulate and define the nursing practice of their staff. Those who favor institutional licensure believe that employers and employees would have more freedom in defining job responsibilities, people would be able to use all their skills developed through both education and experience, and opportunities for advancement would be based on ability.

Those who oppose institutional licensure cite several reasons for their opposition and concerns. They believe that hospitals may be tempted to assign nursing responsibilities to anyone, rather than paying for qualified nurses. They are concerned that standards of educational preparation will vary from one institution to another. They are also concerned about the ability of a nurse to move from one institution to another. If each institution decides the qualifications for licensure, opponents of institutional licensure predict chaos for patients as well as nurses. They say that patients will not know what to expect from nurses in different institutions and that nurses will find it very difficult to move from one institution to another or from one state to another.

Another issue related to licensure has to do with health care workers who are not presently licensed. Medicare regulations reflect the growing concern about the quality of care delivered in nursing homes and other long-term care facilities. As a result, educational requirements for licensure and certification have been proposed. Health care providers have some of the same concerns, and many require that nursing assistants complete an approved program of study before employment. This issue of licensing other health care workers will continue to be debated.

Again, you are in a position to affect the decisions that will be made related to licensure. Since present licensure regulations are based on laws, these regulations can be changed only by changing the law. Keep informed of advantages and disadvantages of various licensure issues, and let your legislators know which position you favor and why.

Nursing Shortage

Many factors have contributed to a nursing shortage. Some of these factors, such as low wages, shift rotations, and lack of respect from employers and physicians, lead to nurses' quitting their profession. Other factors, such as expanded opportunities for women in other fields, an increasing lack of interest in entering a service occupation, and a decrease in the number of young people in this country, affect the number of students enrolling in nursing education programs.

Another factor contributing to a nursing shortage in this country is related to an increasing demand for nurses. Hospitalized patients are acutely ill and require more nursing time than they did in the past. The size of the elderly population has increased rapidly and will continue to do so for the next 20 to 30 years. Meeting the nursing needs of this population requires more nursing time than in the past. Community and home health care and an emphasis on health maintenance offer employment opportunities not previously available to nurses.

Some of the obvious benefits of a nurse shortage are increased wages, more employment opportunities, improved benefits, including tuition assistance with both basic and advanced nursing education, and the potential to bargain for special benefits from your employer. Some of the obvious problems of a nurse shortage is a heavier work load, longer hours, frustration resulting from not having enough time to provide the kind of nursing care you want to provide, and requests from employers to work extra shifts and extra days. These problems contribute to personal stress and "burnout," causing many nurses to leave nursing and thereby compounding the nursing shortage.

The nursing shortage is not going to be resolved in the near future, and is an issue that will directly affect you during your career. You should make every effort to understand how the nursing shortage is now affecting or will affect you and your community and what you can do to offset some of the problems that come with an acute shortage. Getting young people, friends, relatives, and neighbors interested in a career in nursing is a good place to start. Offer to present career information to school, church, and civic groups. Being proud of yourself and what you do often helps others view nursing as a rewarding career. Offering suggestions to your supervisor on how to maximize the efficiency of your nursing team will help you and your colleagues cope with a heavy work load.

Political efforts to resolve the national nursing shortage will no doubt raise many issues that will directly affect you. Keep informed of methods politicians and employers propose. If proposals would jeopardize patient care, voice your objections. Make suggestions and recommendations of your own.

Work Stoppages

A serious question of ethics is raised when nurses or other health care workers strike. Certain occupations, including nursing, fall within the principle of public trust; nurses protect the general health and safety of the public, which, without them, would be vulnerable to illness, injury, or other calamity. Do those whom the public relies on for protection have the right to leave the public unprotected by striking? The question of a nurse's right to strike is an issue that you may have to face during your career.

Health Care Costs

Technological advances, while contributing to improved health care, have contributed to its cost. Dealing with the nursing shortage by increasing salaries increases the cost of health care. Research to find the cause and cure for chronic diseases is very expensive. Building modern health care facilities adds to the cost of health care. The high cost of malpractice insurance also contributes to the increasing cost of health care. Although efforts have been and are being made to control the rising costs of health care, few have been successful.

As the cost of health care escalates, the ability of the patient to pay these costs becomes an increasing financial burden. The cost of care for a catastrophic or chronic illness, such as acquired immune deficiency syndrome (AIDS), birth defects, arthritis, cancer, stroke, or Alzheimer's disease, often exceeds the limits of the patient's health insurance policy and of his ability to pay for his health care. A catastrophic illness is one that is expected to continue for a long period, is costly to treat, requires extensive nursing care and rehabilitation, and depletes the financial resources of the patient and his family.

This issue is currently being addressed by the federal government. Any "catastrophic health insurance" progam that the federal government may develop will have some effect on you. An increase in your personal income tax may be necessary to fund this insurance plan. More people with catastrophic and chronic illnesses may seek medical care, thereby increasing the patient population and exaggerating the nursing shortage. A member of your family who develops a catastrophic illness may, if catastrophic health insurance becomes a reality, not lose his life savings and his home to pay for the cost of health care.

Chemically Impaired Nurses

An issue that will confront you as you begin your career in practical/vocational nursing is that of the chemically impaired nurse. The incidence of drug and alcohol abuse by nurses has increased significantly. Whether or not you personally know a nurse who is addicted to drugs or alcohol, this kind of behavior affects you as well as it does all of nursing. If you work with someone whom you suspect is suffering from an addictive disease, handle the situation with tact and sensitivity. You can accept the person, but you are not expected to accept the addiction. Most large cities have counseling programs specifically designed for members of the health professions. Encourage the person to seek counseling through one of these programs or through other counseling services, before the addiction damages the status of nurses and nursing.

Ethical Issues

Ethical issues will provide many concerns. Chapter 9 reviewed a few ethical issues, but there are many others. The Surgeon General of the United States predicts that 300,000 cases of AIDS will be diagnosed by 1991. The CDC predicts that by 1991 nearly 10 million people will be carrying the AIDS virus. Safely providing nursing care for patients with AIDS is a deep concern for many nurses. Issues related to the quality of life versus the right to die, the right to health care regardless of one's ability to pay, the use of anencephalic newborns as organ donors, surrogate motherhood, and termination of treatment are issues that affect you both as a person and as a nurse.

Learn as much as you can about these and other issues. Look at each issue from your personal point of view and from society's point of view. When you can accept the right of people and society to have opinions different from yours, you will be able to provide nursing care to all your patients, regardless of their personal decisions.

Entry Into Practice

Entry into practice is probably the most important issue facing you as you begin your career in practical/vocational nursing. "Entry into practice" is a term used to imply that there are minimum educational requirements and competencies for entry into the practice of nursing. Although the term itself is not an issue, the way in which the term is used today identifies an issue that has been hotly debated for many years by nurses and nursing organizations around the country.

In 1965 the American Nurses' Association (ANA) published a paper in which the association stated its position on the minimum educational preparation for entry into professional (registered) nursing. This publication stated that the minimum education for professional nurses must be a baccalaureate degree with a major in nursing and that the minimum education for a technical nurse be an associate degree. This 1965 proposal recommended that practical/vocational nursing education be upgraded to beginning-level technical nursing education in community and junior colleges.

The ANA has remained firm in its position on the educational requirements for entry into practice. In 1979 the ANA released another report of a study that again recommended the same two levels of educational preparation for the practice of nursing.

Some of the effects of two levels of nursing education are readily apparent and raise many questions. Where would the hospital nursing school graduate and the practical/vocational nursing school graduate who are already practicing their nursing skills fit into this two-level system? Would they be required to return to school or lose their licenses? What would be the differences between professional and technical nurses? What would be the legal title of each? What licensing examination would be administered?

Other effects of the ANA proposal are not so apparent. What effect would placing all nursing education in colleges and universities have on the cost of nursing education? Would minorities and disadvantaged persons be able to meet the costs of college tuition? Would baccalaureate and associate degree nursing programs have enough space to educate those who wanted to become nurses? Would educational programs be accessible in local communities, or would students have to relocate in order to be enrolled in a nursing program? Are all the nursing needs of all the patients so complex that a college degree must be the minimum preparation?

These are just a few of the questions and issues related to the educational preparation for entry into nursing practice that have divided nurses and nursing for the past 20 to 30 years. Various nursing organizations, health care organizations, and other interested organizations have issued statements outlining their positions on these issues. Some organizations support the proposal; others do not.

Although this issue is not yet resolved, the reality of two levels of educational preparation is much closer than it was in 1965 or even in 1978. What happens to the licensed practical/vocational nurse will depend in large part on how involved each and every licensed practical/vocational nurse is in maintaining career viability. Involvement means that you must let the public know what you do and how well you do it. You must provide the level of nursing care you were taught to deliver. You must inform legislators of the contributions you make in special areas of nursing, such as long-term care. You must also provide facts on how the two levels of entry into practice would affect the nursing shortage. You must join your nursing organizations to provide strength through numbers. You must know the position of your elected officials on this issue and vote accordingly at election time. You must, above all, respect yourself and your chosen career. It is a career that is personally rewarding and vital to the health and welfare of our society. It is a career worth protecting.

In Conclusion

This chapter has presented some of the issues being discussed and debated today. What the future holds is unknown. There will no doubt be new issues and new concerns. Technology will continue to have an impact on how we live our lives and where. Some ethical dilemmas will be resolved, and new ones will develop. The issue of entry into practice will continue to be a major concern. Your only chance of enjoying a long and rewarding career in nursing is to take advantage of every educational opportunity that comes your way and to develop a deep interest in improving the health and comfort of your patients.

Discussion Questions/Learning Activities

1. Review several brochures announcing continuing education programs. How much do these programs cost, where are they held, are credits offered, and what audience are they designed to attract? Would attending any of these programs improve your nursing practice?
2. Prepare a list of states that require continuing education for renewal of the LP/VN license. How many hours are required?

(Continued)

Are the requirements specific or general? (Your librarian can assist you in finding this information in your library.)

3. Write to your state board of nursing and ask for a summary of activities related to mandatory continuing education for license renewal.

4. Is there a shortage of nursing in your geographic area? Information on this question may be available from your local chamber of commerce, your public library, or employers in your area who hire nurses.

5. Find someone in your class who has a point of view opposite yours and debate the right of nurses to go on strike.

6. In addition to the issues discussed in this chapter, what other issues and future concerns can you identify and describe?

7. What emotional response do you have related to the entry-into-practice issue? What activities have you participated in or will you participate in to protect your interests and your career?

8. Take a position on any current issue in nursing and defend it. When appropriate, include facts and figures to support your position.

9. What is your greatest concern for your future as a nurse? What can you do to influence the outcome?

References

Aiken LH: Nursing in the 1980s: Crisis, Opportunities, Challenges. Philadelphia, JB Lippincott, 1982.

Banister E: Contemporary Health Issues. Boston, Jones and Bartlett, 1987.

Bilitski J, Taylor MC (eds): Nursing in the Year Two Thousand. Morgantown, WV, West Virginia University Press, 1984.

Bullough B, Bullough VL, Soukup MC (eds): Nursing Issues and Nursing Strategies for the Eighties. New York, Springer-Verlag, 1983.

Fitzpatrick ML: Prologue to Professionalism. East Norwalk, CT, Appleton & Lange, 1983.

Grippando GM: Nursing Perspectives and Issues. Albany, NY, Delmar, 1986.

Pettengill MM, Young LA: Society in Transition: Impact on Nursing. Indianapolis, IN, Midwest Alliance in Nursing, 1987.

Appendixes

A
Abbreviations Common in Nursing

Abbreviation	Meaning	Abbreviation	Meaning
AA	Alcoholics Anonymous	cc.	cubic centimeter
aa.	of each	CDC	Centers for Disease Control
abd.	abdomen		
ABG	arterial blood gas	cm	centimeter
ADA diet	American Diabetes Association diet	CNS	central nervous system
		CPR	cardiopulmonary resuscitation
ADL	activities of daily living		
		C&S	culture and sensitivity
a.c.	before meals	CSF	cerebrospinal fluid
ad lib.	as much as desired	CV	cardiovascular
AIDS	acquired immune deficiency syndrome	CXR	chest x-ray
		d	day; 24 hours
A/K	above-knee (amputation)	DNR	do not resuscitate
		DOB	date of birth
a.k.a.	also known as	DPT	diptheria-pertussis-tetanus vaccine
AV	atrioventricular		
AWOL	absent without leave	dr	dram
		DWI	driving while intoxicated
b.i.d.	twice a day		
BL = BS	bilateral equal breath sounds	ECG or EKG	electrocardiogram
BM; bm	bowel movement		
BP	blood pressure	EEG	electroencephalogram
BR c̄ BRP	bed rest with bathroom privileges	elix.	elixir
		ENT	ear, nose, throat
BUN	blood urea nitrogen	et	and
C	Celsius, centrigrade, kilocalorie	ETOH	ethyl alcohol
c̄	with	F	Fahrenheit
ca.	about (circa)	FDA	Food and Drug Administration (U.S.)
CAI	computer-assisted instruction		
caps.	capsule	feb.	febrile (fever)
CBC	complete blood count	fld.	fluid

Abbreviation	Meaning	Abbreviation	Meaning
fldext.	fluidextract	NANDA	North American Nursing Diagnosis Association
GI	gastrointestinal		
Gm; gm	gram	NIDDM	non-insulin-dependent diabetes mellitus
gr	grain		
Gtt; gtt	drop		
G/W	glucose in water		
Gyn	gynecology	NPN	nonprotein nitrogen
		NPO	nothing by mouth
h	hour	NVD	nausea, vomiting, and diarrhea
hct.	hematocrit		
Hgb	hemoglobin		
H_2O	water	o.d.	once daily
H_2O_2	peroxide	o.d.	right eye
HPI	history of present illness	oob	out of bed
		OOP	out on pass
h.s.	at bedtime	os	mouth
↑ICP	increased intracranial pressure	o.s.	left eye
		o.u.	both eyes
IDDM	insulin-dependent diabetes mellitus	oz.	ounce
I.M.	intramuscularly	PBI	protein-bound iodine
IPPB	intermittent positive-pressure breathing	p.c.	after meals
		PCO_2	partial pressure of carbon dioxide
IQ	intelligence quotient	per	through; by
IUD	intrauterine device	pH	hydrogen ion concentration
I.V.	intravenously		
kg	kilogram	PMH	past medical history
KUB	kidneys, ureters, and bladder		
KVO	keep vein open	p.o.	by mouth
		PO_2	partial pressure of oxygen
L	liter		
lab	laboratory	p.r.n.	as needed
lb.	pound	pt.	pint; patient
LMP	last menstrual period	q.	every
LPM	liters per minute	q.d.	every day
liq.	liquid	q.h.	every hour
m	meter	q.2h.	every 2 hours
mcg	microgram	q.3h.	every 3 hours
mg	milligram	q.i.d.	4 times a day
ml	milliliter	q.o.d.	every other day
mEq	milliequivalent	q.s.	quantity sufficient
Na	sodium; salt	qt.	quart

Abbreviation	Meaning	Abbreviation	Meaning
rad	radiation absorbed dose	tr.	tincture
resp.	respiration	trach	tracheotomy
Rh	rhesus blood factor	U	unit
R/O	rule out	USP	United States Pharmacopeia
Rx	take	UV	ultraviolet
s̄	without	WBC	white blood cell count
SIDS	sudden infant death syndrome	Wt.	weight
S.C. or sc	subcutaneously	>	greater than
s.o.s.	if necessary	<	less than
sp. frumenti	whiskey	=	equal to
		≠	not equal
sp. gr.	specific gravity	♂	male
ss	one half	♀	female
stat	immediately	oz, ℥	ounce
syr.	syrup	dr ap, ʒ	dram
tab.	tablet	min, ♏	minim
t.i.d.	3 times a day	:	ratio, "is to"
top.	topically	::	equality between ratios; "as"
TPR	temperature, pulse, respiration	°	degree

B
Common Sexually Transmitted Diseases

Disease	Usual Time from Contact to First Symptoms	Usual Symptoms	Complications
Gonorrhea Cause: bacterium	2-10 days; sometimes 30 days	Local, genital discharge, pain; often no symptoms in men; usually no symptoms in women	Pelvic inflammatory disease, sterility, arthritis, blindness, eye infection in newborns
Syphilis Cause: spirochete	3-5 weeks; Average 21 days	First stage: painless pimple that disappears without treatment on genitals, fingers, lips, breast; second stage: rash, fever, flu-like illness; latent stage: none	Brain damage, insanity, paralysis, heart disease, death, damage to skin, bones, eyes, liver, teeth of fetus and newborns
Genital Herpes Cause: virus	About 1 week	Swollen, tender, painful blisters on genitals	Strong evidence linking infection to cervical cancer; severe central nervous system damage or death in infants infected during birth
Nonspecific Vaginitis Cause: (?) bacterium	1-2 weeks	Gray offensive vaginal discharge, usually no itching	Medical complications unknown
Nonspecific Urethritis Cause: Chlamydia	1-3 weeks	Penile discharge, frequent urination; usually no itching	Pelvic inflammatory disease in women, possible eye infections or pneumonia in newborns
Trichomonas Cause: protozoon	1-4 weeks	Discharge, intense itching, burning and redness of genitals and thighs; painful intercourse; usually no symptoms in men	Gland infections in females, prostatitis in men
Monilia Cause: fungus	Varies	Thick, cheesy, offensive vaginal discharge; itching, skin irritation; usually no symptoms in men	Seconday infections by bacteria; mouth and throat infections of newborn
Venereal Warts Cause: virus	Up to 2 months	Local irritation, itching	Highly contagious; can spread enough to block vaginal opening
Pediculosis Pubis Cause: louse	4-5 weeks	Intense itching, pinhead blood spots on underwear; small eggs or nits on pubic hair	No medical complications
Scabies Cause: itch mite	4-6 weeks	Severe nighttime itching, raised gray lines in skin where mite burrows	May infest elbows, hands, breasts, and buttocks as well as genitals
AIDS (acquired immune deficiency syndrome)	Not established. May be 3 months to 2 yrs.	Lymph gland swelling (swollen glands), flu-like illness of long duration, purplish discolorations on arms and legs, unexplained weight loss, persistent cough, loss of appetite	Kaposi's sarcoma (a form of cancer), pneumonia, various other life-threatening infections, death

C
Stress Management Techniques

The following techniques can be taught to provide an individual with an opportunity to control his response to stressors and thus in turn increase his ability to manage stress constructively. Suggested readings are listed at the end to provide more specific information.

Progressive Relaxation Technique

Progressive relaxation is a self-taught or instructed exercise that involves learning to constrict and relax muscle groups in a systematic way, beginning with the face and finishing with the feet. This exercise may be combined with breathing exercises that focus on inner body processes. It usually takes 15 to 30 minutes and may be accompanied by a taped instruction that directs the person concerning the sequence of muscles to be relaxed.

1. Wear loose clothing; remove glasses and shoes
2. Sit or recline in a comfortable position with neck and knees supported; avoid lying completely flat
3. Begin with slow, rhythmic breathing
   a. Close your eyes or stare at a spot and take in a slow deep breath
   b. Exhale the breath slowly
4. Continue rhythmic breathing at a slow steady pace and feel the tension leaving your body with each breath
5. Begin progressive relaxation of muscle groups
   a. Breathe in and tense (tighten) your muscles and then relax the muscles as you breathe out
   b. Suggested order for tension-relaxation cycle (with tension technique in parenthesis)
      Face, jaw, mouth (squint eyes, wrinkle brow)
      Neck (pull chin to neck)
      Right hand (make a fist)
      Right arm (bend elbow in tightly)
      Left hand (make a fist)
      Left arm (bend elbow in tightly)
      Back, shoulders, chest (shrug shoulders up tightly)
      Abdomen (pull stomach in and bear down on chair)

From Carpenito L: Nursing Diagnosis: Application to Clinical Practice. Philadelphia, JB Lippincott, 1983, pp 522–524.

> Right upper leg (push leg down)
> Right lower leg and foot (point toes toward body)
> Left upper leg (push leg down)
> Left lower leg and foot (point toes toward body)

6. Practice technique slowly
7. End relaxation session when you are ready by counting to three, inhaling deeply, and saying, "I am relaxed"

Self-coaching

Self-coaching is a procedure to decrease anxiety by understanding one's own signs of anxiety (such as increased heart rate or sweaty palms) and then coaching oneself to relax.

For example, "I am upset about this situation but I can control how anxious I get. I will take things one step at a time, and I won't focus on my fear. I'll think about what I must do to finish this task. The situation will not be forever. I can manage until it is over. I'll focus on taking slow deep breaths."

Thought Stopping

Thought stopping is a self-directed behavioral procedure learned to gain control of self-defeating thoughts. Through repeated systematic practice, a person does the following:

1. Says "Stop" when a self-defeating thought crosses the mind (e.g., "I'm not smart enough" or "I'm not a good nurse")
2. Allows a brief period—15 to 30 seconds—of conscious relaxation (because of an increased focus on negative thoughts, it may seem at first that self-defeating thoughts increase; however, eventually the self-defeating thoughts will decrease).

Assertive Behavior

Assertive behavior is the open, honest, empathetic sharing of your opinions, desires, and feelings. Assertiveness is not a magical acquisition but a learned behavioral skill. Assertive persons do not allow others to take advantage of them and thus are not victims. Assertive behavior is not domineering but remains controlled and non-aggressive. An assertive person

> Does not hurt others
> Does not wait for things to get better
> Does not invite victimization
> Listens attentively to the desires and feelings of others
> Takes the initiative to make relationships better
> Remains in control or uses silences as an alternative
> Examines all the risks involved before asserting
> Examines personal responsibilities in each situation before asserting

Refer to suggested readings for specific techniques or participate in an assertiveness training course led by a competent instructor. Assertive behavior is best learned slowly in several sessions rather than in one lengthy session or workshop.

Guided Imagery

This technique is the purposeful use of one's imagination in a specific way to achieve relaxation and control. The person concentrates on the image and pictures himself involved in the scene. The following is an example of the technique.

1. Discuss with person an image he has experienced that is pleasurable and relaxing to him, such as

    Lying on a warm beach

    Feeling a cool wave of water

    Floating on a raft

    Watching the sun set

2. Choose a scene that will involve at least two senses
3. Begin with rhythmic breathing and progressive relaxation
4. Have person travel mentally to the scene
5. Have the person slowly experience the scene; how does it look? sound? smell? feel? taste?
6. Practice the imagery
    a. Suggest tape-recording the imagined experience to assist with the technique
    b. Practice the technique alone to reduce feelings of embarrassment
7. End the imagery technique by counting to three and saying, "I am relaxed" (if the person does not utilize a specific ending, he may become drowsy and fall asleep, which defeats the purpose of the technique)

Suggested Readings

Alberti RE, Emmons L: Your Perfect Right: A Guide to Assertive Behavior, 2nd ed. San Luis Obispo, CA, Impact, 1974

Benson H: The Relaxation Response. New York, Avon Books, 1976

Bloom L, Coburn K, Pearlman J: The New Assertive Woman. New York, Dell, 1976

Chenevert M: Special Techniques in Assertiveness Training for Women in the Health Professions, 3rd ed. St. Louis, CV Mosby, 1987

Gridano D, Everly G: Controlling Stress and Tension. Englewood Cliffs, NJ, Prentice-Hall, 1979

Herman S: Becoming Assertive: A Guide for Nurses. New York, D Van Nostrand, 1978

McCaffery M: Nursing Management of the Patient with Pain, 2nd ed. Philadelphia, JB Lippincott, 1979 (especially Chapter 10, Imagery; Chapter 9, Relaxation)

D

Nursing Practice Standards for the Licensed Practical/Vocational Nurse

Preface

The Standards replace the "Statement of Functions and Qualifications" as approved by the Executive Board of the National Federation of Licensed Practical Nurses in June 1970 and revised in April 1972 and were developed and adopted by the NFLPN to provide a basic model whereby the quality of health service and nursing care given by LP/VNs may be measured and evaluated.

These nursing practice standards are applicable in any practice setting. The degree to which individual standards are applied will vary according to the individual needs of the patient, the type of health care agency or services and the community resources.

The scope of licensed practical nursing has extended into specialized nursing services. Therefore, specialized fields of nursing are included in this document.

The Code for Licensed Practical/Vocational Nurses

The Code adopted by NFLPN in 1961 and revised in 1979 provided a motivation for establishing and elevating professional standards. Each LP/VN, upon entering the profession, inherits the responsibility to adhere to the standards of ethical practice and conduct as set forth in this Code.

1. Know the scope of maximum utilization of the LP/VN as specified by the nursing practice act and function within this scope.
2. Safeguard the confidential information acquired from any source about the patient.
3. Provide health care to all patients regardless of race, creed, cultural background, disease, or lifestyle.
4. Refuse to give endorsement to the sale and promotion of commercial products or services.

5. Uphold the highest standards in personal appearance, language, dress, and demeanor.
6. Stay informed about issues affecting the practice of nursing and delivery of health care and, where appropriate, participate in government and policy decisions.
7. Accept the responsibility for safe nursing by keeping oneself mentally and physically fit and educationally prepared to practice.
8. Accept responsibility for membership in NFLPN and participate in its efforts to maintain the established standards of nursing practice and employment policies conducive to quality patient care.

Introductory Statement

Definition

Practical/Vocational nursing means the performance for compensation of authorized acts of nursing which utilize specialized knowledge and skills and which meet the health needs of people in a variety of settings under the direction of qualified health professionals.

Scope

Practical/Vocational nursing comprises the common core of nursing and, therefore, is a valid entry into the nursing profession.

Opportunities exist for practicing in a milieu where different professions unite their particular skills in a team effort for one common objective—to preserve or improve an individual patient's functioning.

Opportunities also exist for upward mobility within the profession through academic education and for lateral expansion of knowledge and expertise through both academic and continuing education.

Standards

Education

The Licensed Practical/Vocational Nurse

1. Shall complete a formal education program in practical nursing approved by the appropriate nursing authority in a state.
2. Shall successfully pass the National State Board Examination for Licensed Practical Nurses.
3. Shall participate in initial orientation within the employing institution.

Legal/Ethical Status

The Licensed Practical/Vocational Nurse

1. Shall hold a current license to practice nursing as an LP/VN in accordance with the law of the state wherein employed.
2. Shall know the scope of nursing practice authorized by the Nursing Practice Act in the state wherein employed.
3. Shall have a personal commitment to fulfill the legal responsibilities inherent in good nursing practice.
4. Shall take responsible actions in situations wherein there is unprofessional conduct by a peer or other health care provider.
5. Shall recognize and have a commitment to meet the ethical and moral obligations of the practice of nursing.
6. Shall not accept or perform professional responsibilities which the individual knows (s)he is not competent to perform.

Practice

The Licensed Practical/Vocational Nurse

1. Shall accept assigned responsibilities as an accountable member of the health care team.
2. Shall function within the limits of educational preparation and experience as related to the assigned duties.
3. Shall function with other members of the health care team in promoting and maintaining health, preventing disease and disability, caring for and rehabilitating individuals who are experiencing altered health state, and to contribute to the patients ultimate quality of life until death.
4. Shall know and utilize the nursing process in planning, implementing, and evaluating health services and nursing care to the individual patient or group.
   a. Planning: The planning of nursing includes:
      1. assessment of health status of the individual patient, the family and community groups
      2. an analysis of the information gained from assessment
      3. the identification of health goals.
   b. Implementation: The plan for nursing care is implemented to achieve the stated goals and includes:
      1. observing, recording and reporting significant changes which requires intervention or different goals
      2. application of nursing knowledge and skills to promote and maintain health, to prevent disease and disability and to optimize functional capabilities of an individual patient
      3. assisting the patient and family with activities of daily living and encouraging self-care as appropriate
      4. carry out therapeutic regimens and protocols prescribed by an RN, physician, or other persons authorized by state law.

c. Evaluations: The plan for nursing care and its implementations are evaluated to measure the progress toward the stated goals and will include appropriate persons and/or groups to determine:
   1. the relevancy of current goals in relation to the progress of the individual patient
   2. the involvement of the recipients of care in the evaluation process
   3. the quality of the nursing action in the implementation of the plan
   4. a re-ordering of priorities or new goal setting in the care plan.
5. Shall participate in peer review and other evaluation processes.
6. Shall participate in the development of policies concerning the health and nursing needs of society and in the roles and functions of the LP/VN.

Continuing Education

The Licensed Practical/Vocational Nurse

1. Shall be responsible for maintaining the highest possible level of professional competence at all times.
2. Shall periodically reassess career goals and select continuing education activities which will help to achieve these goals.
3. Shall take advantage of continuing education opportunities which will lead to personal growth and professional development.
4. Shall seek and participate in continuing education activities which are approved for credit by the nationally accepted and recognized CEU.

Specialized Nursing Practice

The Licensed Practical/Vocational Nurse

1. Shall have had at least one year's experience in nursing at the staff level.
2. Shall present personal qualifications that are indicative of potential abilities for practice in the chosen specialized nursing area.
3. Shall present evidence of completion of a program or course that is approved by an appropriate agency to provide the knowledge and skills necessary for effective nursing services in the specialized field.
4. Shall meet all of the standards of practice as set forth in this document.

Glossary

Authorized (acts of nursing)—legalized through State Nurse Practice Acts

CEU—continuing education unit

Lateral Expansion of Knowledge—extension of the basic core of information learned in the school of practical nursing.

Peer Review—evaluation of performance on the job by other LP/VNs.

Specialized Nursing Practice—a restricted field of nursing in which a person is particularly skilled and has specific knowledge.

Therapeutic Regimens—regulated plans designed to bring about effective treatment of disease.

Upward Mobility—change of career goal, e.g., Licensed Practical/Vocational Nurse to Registered Nurse.

LP/VN—The LPN is the same as the LVN in California and Texas.

Milieu—Environment and surroundings.

Revised 1987

E
NAPNES Standards of Practice for Licensed Practical/Vocational Nurses

The LP/VN Provides Individual and Family-Centered Nursing Care

A. Utilize principles of nursing process in meeting specific patient needs of patients of all ages in the areas of:
1. Safety
2. Hygiene
3. Nutrition
4. Medication
5. Elimination
6. Psycho-social and cultural
7. Respiratory needs

B. Utilize appropriate knowledge, skills and abilities in providing safe, competent care.

C. Utilize principles of crisis intervention in maintaining safety and making appropriate referrals when necessary.

D. Utilize effective communication skills.
1. Communicate effectively with patients, family members of the health team, and significant others.
2. Maintain appropriate written documentation

E. Provide appropriate health teaching to patients and significant others in the areas of:
1. Maintenance of wellness
2. Rehabilitation
3. Utilization of community resources

F. Serves as a patient advocate:
1. Protect patient rights
2. Consult with appropriate others when necessary

Reprinted with permission of the National Association for Practical Nurse Education and Service. Copyright 1985.

The LP/VN Fulfills the Professional Responsibilities of the Practical/Vocational Nurse. The LP/VN shall:

A. Know and apply the ethical principles underlying the profession.
B. Know and follow the appropriate professional and legal requirements.
C. Follow the policies and procedures of the employing institution.
D. Cooperate and collaborate with all members of the health care team to meet the needs of family-centered nursing care.
E. Demonstrate accountability for his/her nursing actions.
F. Maintain currency in terms of knowledge and skills in the area of employment.

Adopted 1985

F
Directory of Nursing and Health-Related Organizations

This appendix is divided into five parts. Part I is a listing of state boards of nursing alphabetically by state; Part II is a listing of Canadian associations and boards of nursing; Part III is a list of national practical/vocational nursing organizations; Part IV lists the addresses of the state affiliates of the National Association for Practical Nurse Education and Service; and Part V is a listing of additional organizations of particular interest to practical nurses.

(Note: These addresses were current as of June-December 1987.)

Part I   *State Boards of Nursing*

Alabama Board of Nursing
500 Eastern Blvd.,
One/East Building, Suite 203
Montgomery, Alabama 36117
Tel: 205/261-4060
Shirley Dykes, Executive Officer

Alaska Board of Nursing
Division of Occupational Licensing
3601 C St., Suite 722
Anchorage, Alaska 99503
Tel: 907/561-2878
Gail M. McGuill, Executive Secretary

American Samoa Health Service
Regulatory Board
Pago Pago, American Samoa 96799
Tel: 684/633-1222 ext. 206
Elizabeth B.U. Malae, Executive Secretary

Arizona State Board of Nursing
5050 N. 19th Ave.
Suite 103
Phoenix, Arizona 85015
Tel: 602/255-5092
Floretta Awe, Acting Executive Director

Arkansas State Board of Nursing
University Towers Building
West 12th St. & University Ave., Suite 800
Little Rock, Arkansas 72204
Tel: 501/371-2751
June Garner, Executive Director

California Board of Vocational Nurse
  and Psychiatric Technician Examiners
1020 N St., Room 406
Sacramento, California 95814
Tel: 916/323-2168
Billie Haynes, Executive Officer

Colorado Board of Nursing
State Services Building, Room 132
1525 Sherman St.
Denver, Colorado 80203
Tel: 303/866-2871
Karen Brumley, Program Administrator

Connecticut Board of Examiners for
  Nursing
150 Washington St.
Hartford, Connecticut 06106
Tel: 203/566-1041
Marie T. Hilliard, Executive Officer

District of Columbia
Board of Nursing
614 H. St., N.W.
Washington, DC 20001
Tel: 202/727-7468
Barbara Hagans, Contact Person

Delaware Board of Nursing
Margaret O'Neill Building
P.O. Box 1401
Dover, Delaware ;19901
Tel: 202/736-4752
Rosalee J. Seymour, Executive Director

Florida Board of Nursing
111 Coastline Dr., East
Jacksonville, Florida 32202
Tel: 904/359-6331
Judie K. Ritter, Executive Director

Georgia State Board of Licensed
   Practical Nurses
166 Pryor St., S.W.
Atlanta, Georgia 30303
Tel: 404/656-3921
Patricia N. Swann, Executive Director

Guam Board of Nurse Examiners
P.O. Box 2816
Agana, Guam 96910
Tel: 671/734-4813
Teofila P. Cruz, Nurse Examiner
   Administrator

Hawaii Board of Nursing
P.O. Box 3469
Honolulu, Hawaii 96801
Tel: 808/548-3086
Jerold Sakoda, Executive Secretary

Idaho Board of Nursing
500 South 10th St.
Suite 102
Boise, Idaho 83720
Tel: 208/334-3110
Phyllis T. Sheridan, Executive Director

Illinois Department of Registration and
   Education
320 West Washington St.
3rd Floor
Springfield, Illinois 62786

Tel: 217/782-4386
Judy A. Otto, Nursing Education
   Coordinator

Indiana State Board of Nursing
Health Professions Bureau
One American Square
Suite 1020, Box 82067
Indianapolis, Indiana 46282-0004
Tel: 317/232-2960
Larry Sage, Board Administrator

Iowa Board of Nursing
Executive Hills East
1223 East Court
Des Moines, Iowa 50319
Tel: 515/281-3256
Ann E. Mowery, Executive Director

Kansas Board of Nursing
Landon State Office Building
900 S. W. Jackson, Suite 551 S
Topeka, Kansas 66612-1256
Tel: 913/296-4929
Lois Rich Scibetta, Executive
   Administrator

Kentucky Board of Nursing
4010 Dupont Circle
Suite 430
Louisville, Kentucky 40207
Tel: 502/897-5143
Sharon M. Weisenbeck, Executive
   Director

Louisiana State Board of Practical Nurse
   Examiners
1440 Canal St.
Suite 2010
New Orleans, Louisiana 70112
Tel: 504/568-6480
Terry L. DeMarcay, Executive Director

Maine State Board of Nursing
295 Water St.
Augusta, Maine 04330
Tel: 207/289-5324
Jean C. Caron, Executive Director

Maryland Board of Examiners for Nurses
201 West Preston St.
Baltimore, Maryland 21201

Tel: 301/225-5880

Donna M. Dorsey, Executive Director

Massachusetts Board of Registration in
  Nursing
Everett Saltonslahl Building
100 Cambridge St., Room 1519
Boston, Massachusetts 02202
Tel: 617/727-7393
Mary H. Snodgrass, Executive Secrtary

Michigan Board of Nursing
Ottowa Towers North
611 West Ottawa
P.O. Box 30018
Lansing, Michigan 48909
Tel: 517/373-1600
Elizabeth Jensen, Nursing Consultant

Minnesota Board of Nursing
2700 University Ave. W.
No. 108
St. Paul, Minnesota 55114
Tel: 612/642-0567
Joyce M. Schowalter, Executive Director

Mississippi Board of Nursing
135 Bounds St.
Suite 101
Jackson, Mississippi 39206
Tel: 601/354-7349
Marcella McKay, Executive Director

Missouri State Board of Nursing
P.O. Box 656
3523 N. Ten Mile Dr.
Jefferson City, Missouri 65102
Tel: 314/751-2334, ext. 141
Florence McGuire, Executive Director

Montana State Board of N. rsing
1424 9th Ave.
Helena, Montana 59620-0407
Tel: 406/444-4279
Phyllis McDonald, Executive Secretary

Bureau of Examining Boards
Nebraska Department of Health
P.O. Box 95007
Lincoln, Nebraska 68509
Tel: 402/471-2001
Eunice Casey, Associate Director

Nevada State Board of Nursing
1281 Terminal Way
Suite 116
Reno, Nevada 89502
Tel: 702/786-2778
Volanda Burress, Executive Director

New Hampshire Board of Nursing
Health and Welfare Building
6 Hazen Dr.
Concord, New Hampshire 03301-6527
Tel: 603/271-2323
Doris Nay, Executive Director

New Jersey Board of Nursing
1100 Raymond Blvd., Room 319
Newark, New Jersey 07102
Tel: 201/648-2570
Sr. Teresa Harris, Executive Director

New Mexico Board of Nursing
4125 Carlisle N.E.
Albuquerque, New Mexico 87107
Tel.: 505/841-6524 ext. 28
Nancy Twigg, Executive Director

New York State Board for Nursing
State Education Department
Cultural Education Center, Room 3013
Albany, New York 12230
Tel: 518/474-3843
Gail Rosettie, Nursing Education
  Supervisor

North Carolina Board of Nursing
P.O. Box 2129
Raleigh, North Carolina 27602
Tel: 919/828-0740
Carol A. Osman, Executive Director

North Dakota Board of Nursing
Kirkwood Office Tower, Suite 504
7th St. South & Arbor Ave.
Bismarck, North Dakota 58501
Tel: 701/224-2974
Karen Macdonald, Executive Director

Ohio Board of Nursing Education and
Nurse Registration
65 South Front St., Suite 509
Columbus, Ohio 43266-0316
Tel: 614/466-3947
Rosa Lee Weinert, Executive Secretary

Oklahoma Board of Nurse Registration
and Education
2915 N. Classen Blvd.
Suite 524
Oklahoma City, Oklahoma 73106
Tel: 405/525-2076
Sulinda Moffett, Executive Director

Oregon State Board of Nursing
1400 S. W. Fifth Ave., Room 904
Portland, Oregon 97201
Tel: 503/229-5653
Dorothy J. Davy, Executive Director

Pennsylvania Board of Nursing
P.O. Box 2649
Harrisburg, Pennsylvania 17105-2649
Tel: 717/783-7146
Miriam H. Limo, Executive Secretary

Rhode Island Board of Nurse
    Registration & Nurse Education
Cannon Health Building
75 Davis St., Room 104
Providence, Rhode Island 02908-2488
Tel: 401/277-2827
Bertha Mugurdichian, Executive
    Secretary

State Board of Nursing for South Carolina
1777 St. Julian Place, Suite 102
Columbia, South Carolina 29204-2488
Tel: 803/737-3800
Renatta Loquist, Executive Director

South Dakota Board of Nursing
304 S. Phillips Ave., Suite 205
Sioux Falls, South Dakota 57102
Tel: 605/334-1243
Carol A. Stuart, Executive Secretary

Tennessee State Board of Nursing
283 Plus Park Blvd.
Nashville, Tennessee 37217
Tel: 615/367-6232
Elizabeth Lund, Executive Director

Texas Board of Vocational Nurse
    Examiners
1300 East Anderson Lane
Building C, Suite 285
Austin, Texas 78752
Tel: 512/835-2071
Joyce A. Hammer, Executive Director

Utah State Board of Nursing
Heber Wells Building, 4th Floor
160 East 300 South
Salt Lake City, Utah 84145
Tel: 801/530-6628
Ann G. Petersen, Executive Secretary

Vermont State Board of Nursing
Redstone Building
26 Terrace St.
Montpelier, Vermont 05602
Tel: 802/828-2396
Lynn Blake Hardee, Executive Director

Virgin Islands Board of Nurse Licensure
P.O. Box 7309
St. Thomas, Virgin Islands 00801
Tel: 809/774-9000, ext. 132
June Adams, Chairperson

Virginia State Board of Nursing
1601 Rolling Hills Dr.
Richmond, Virginia 23229-5005
Tel: 804/662-9909
Corinne F. Dorsey, Executive Secretary

Washington State Board of Practical
    Nursing
P.O. Box 9649
Olympia, Washington 98504
Tel: 206/586-1923
Susan L. Boots, Executive Secretary

West Virginia State Board of Examiners
    for Practical Nurses
922 Quarrier St.
Embleton Building, Suite 506
Charleston, West Virginia 25301
Tel: 304/348-3572
Nancy R. Wilson, Executive Secretary

Wisconsin Bureau of Health Professions
1400 East Washington Ave.
P.O. Box 8935
Madison, Wisconsin 53708-8935
Tel: 608/266-3735
Ramona Weakland Warden, Director

Wyoming State Board of Nursing
Barrett Building, 4th Floor
2301 Central Ave.
Cheyenne, Wyoming 82002
Tel: 307/777-7601
Joan Bouchard, Executive Director

Part II
Canadian Associations and Boards of Nursing

Alberta Nursing Assistants Registration
Board
10030 107th St., 8th Floor
Edmonton, Alberta T5J 3E4

British Columbia Council of Practical
Nurses
3405 Willingdon Ave.
Burnaby, British Columbia V5G 3H4

Manitoba Association of Licensed
Practical Nurses
1-120 Marion
Winnipeg, Manitoba R2H OT4

Association of New Brunswick
Registered Nursing Assistants
39 Coventry Crescent
Fredericton, New Brunswick E3B 4P4

Nova Scotia Board of Registration for
Nursing Assistants
5614 Fenwick St.
Halifax, Nova Scotia B3H 1P9

Prince Edward Island Licensed Nursing
Assistants Association
P.O. Box 1253
Charlottetown, Prince Edward Island
C1A 7M8

Professional Corporation of Nursing
Assistants of Quebec
1980 Sherbrook West
Room 920
Montreal, Quebec H3H 1E8

Part III National Practical/Vocational
Nursing Organizations

National Association for Practical Nurse
Education and Service
1400 Springs Street
Suite 310
Silver Springs, Maryland 20910
John Word, Executive Director

National Federation of Practical
Nursing, Inc.
P.O. Box 18088
3948 Browning Place
Suite 205
Raleigh, North Carolina 27619
Tel: 919/781-4791
David Kesterson, Executive Director

Part IV NAPNES State Affiliates

Licensed Practical Nurses
Association of Alabama
P.O. Box 1144
Vernon, Alabama 35592

Arizona Federation of Licensed Practical
Nurses
606 West Ajo Way
Tucson, Arizona 85713

Arkansas Licensed Practical Nurse
Association
Commercial Warehouse No. 4

1800 East Roosevelt Rd.
Little Rock, Arkansas 72206

Delaware Licensed Practical Nurse
Association
3301 North Market St.
Wilmington, Delaware 19802

Licensed Practical Nurses Association of
District of Columbia
226 Rhode Island Ave., N.W.
Washington, DC 20001

Florida Licensed Practical Nurse
Association
218 West Lawson Dr.
Auburndale, Florida 33823

Georgia Licensed Practical Nurses
Association
699 Willoughby Way, N.E.
Atlanta, Georgia 30312

Licensed Practical Nurses Association of
Louisiana
3604 Virgil Blvd.
New Orleans, Louisiana 70122

Michigan Licensed Practical Nurses
Association
5900 Executive Dr.
Lansing, Michigan 48911

Mississippi Federation of Licensed
Practical Nurses
No. 308 May Building, Washington Ave.
Greenville, Mississippi 38701

Missouri State Association of Licensed
Practical Nurses
125 W. Dunklin
Suite 15
Jefferson City, Missouri 65101

Licensed Practical Nurses Association of
New Jersey
1811 Springfield Ave.
Maplewood, New Jersey 07040

Licensed Practical Nurses Association of
Ohio
1310 St. Paris Rd.
Springfield, Ohio 45504

Licensed Practical Nurses Association of
Pennsylvania
13 North Progress Ave.
Progress Plaza
Harrisburg, Pennsylvania 17109

Federacion de Enfermeria Practica de
Puerto Rico, Inc.
Box 7745
Bo. Obrero Station
Santurce, Puerto Rico 00916

South Dakota Licensed Practical Nurse
Association
307 8th Ave., S.W.
Aberdeen, South Dakota 57401

Licensed Practical Nurses Association of
Utah
1744 Alfred Dr.
Layton, Utah 84041

Licensed Practical Nurses Association of
Vermont
P.O. Box 468
Randolph, Vermont 05060

Virgin Islands Licensed Practical Nurses
Association
P.O. Box 7943
Sunny Isles
St. Croix, Virgin Islands 00820

Licensed Practical Nurses Association of
Washington State
156 Denny Way
Seattle, Washington 98109

Part V   Other Organizations

American Hospital Association
840 N. Lake Shore Dr.
Chicago, Illinois 60611

American Nurses' Association
2420 Pershing Rd.
Kansas City, Missouri 64108
Tel: 816/474-5720

American Red Cross
17th and D Sts., N.W.
Washington, DC 20006
Tel: 202/737-8300

American Vocational Association
1410 King St.
Alexandria, Virginia 22314

Army Nurse Corps
Office of the Surgeon General
Department of the Army
5111 Leesburg Pike
Falls Church, Virginia 22031-3258
Tel: 202-756-0045

Catholic Health Association of the
United States
4455 Woodson Rd.
St. Louis, Missouri 63134

Federation for Accessible Nursing
Education and Licensure
P.O. Box 22417
Seattle, Washington 98122
Lorraine Sherk, President

Health Occupations Students of America
National Headquarters
4108 Amon Carter Blvd.
Suite 202
Fort Worth, Texas 76155
1-800/321-HOSA

National Council of State Boards of
Nursing
625 North Michigan Ave.
Suite 1544
Chicago, Illinois 60611
Tel: 312/787-6555

National League for Nursing
10 Columbus Circle
New York, New York 10019
Tel: 212/582-1022

National Nurses Society on Addictions
2506 Gross Point Rd.
Evanston, Illinois 60201
Tel: 312/475-7300
Ann Solari-Twadell, President

Nurses Coalition for Action in Politics
Suite 200
1101 14th St., N.W.
Washington, DC 20005

World Health Organization
Avenue Appia
1211 Geneva 27, Switzerland

G
Approved Nursing Diagnoses, North American Nursing Diagnosis Association, June (1988)

Activity intolerance
Activity intolerance, potential
Adjustment, impaired
Airway clearance, ineffective
Anxiety
Aspiration, potential for
Body temperature, altered, potential
Bowel elimination, altered: Constipation
   Colonic constipation
   Perceived constipation
Bowel elimination, altered: Diarrhea
Bowel elimination, altered:
   Incontinence
Breastfeeding, ineffective
Breathing pattern, ineffective
Cardiac output, altered: Decreased
   (specify)
Comfort, altered: Pain
Comfort, altered: Chronic pain
Communication, impaired: Verbal
Coping, family: Potential for growth
Coping, ineffective, family:
   Compromised
Coping, ineffective, family: Disabling
Coping, ineffective, individual
   Defensive coping
   Ineffective denial
Decisional conflict (specify)
Disuse syndrome, potential for
Diversional activity, deficit
Dysreflexia
Family process, altered
Fatigue
Fear
Fluid volume excess

Fluid volume deficit, actual
Fluid volume deficit, potential
Gas exchange, impaired
Grieving, anticipatory
Grieving, dysfunctional
Growth and development, altered
Health maintenance, altered
Health-seeking behaviors (specify)
Home maintenance, impaired
Hopelessness
Hyperthermia
Hypothermia
Incontinence, functional
Incontinence, reflex
Incontinence, stress
Incontinence, total
Incontinence, urge
Infection, potential for
Injury, potential for (specify):
   suffocation, poisoning, trauma
Knowledge deficit (specify)
Mobility, impaired physical
Noncompliance (specify)
Nutrition, altered: Less than body
   requirements
Nutrition, altered: More than body
   requirements
Nutrition, altered: Potential for more
   than body requirements
Oral mucous membrane, altered
Parental role conflict
Parenting, altered: Actual
Parenting, altered: Potential
Post trauma response
Powerlessness

Rape trauma syndrome
Role performance, altered
Self-care deficit: Feeding, bathing/
    hygiene, dressing/grooming, toileting
Self-concept, disturbance in body image,
    self-esteem, role performance,
    personal identity
Self-esteem disturbance
    Chronic low self-esteem
    Situational low self-esteem
Sensory/perceptual alteration: Visual,
    auditory, kinesthetic, gustatory,
    tactile, olfactory
Sexual dysfunction
Sexuality patterns, altered
Skin integrity, impaired: Actual
Skin integrity, impaired: Potential

Sleep pattern disturbance
Social interaction, impaired
Social isolation
Spiritual distress (distress of the human
    spirit)
Swallowing, impaired
Thermoregulation, ineffective
Thought processes, altered
Tissue integrity, impaired
Tissue perfusion, altered: Cerebral,
    cardiopulmonary, renal,
    gastrointestinal, peripheral
Unilateral neglect
Urinary elimination, altered patterns
Urinary retention
Violence, potential for: Self-directed or
    directed at others

H
A Patient's Bill of Rights

The American Hospital Association presents a Patient's Bill of Rights with the expectation that observance of these rights will contribute to more effective patient care and greater satisfaction for the patient, his physician, and the hospital organization. Further, the Association presents these rights in the expectation that they will be supported by the hospital on behalf of its patients, as an integral part of the healing process. It is recognized that a personal relationship between the physician and the patient is essential for the provision of proper medical care. The traditional physician-patient relationship takes on a new dimension when care is rendered within an organizational structure. Legal precedent has established that the institution itself also has a responsibility to the patient. It is in recognition of these factors that these rights are affirmed.

1. The patient has the right to considerate and respectful care.
2. The patient has the right to obtain from his physician complete current information concerning his diagnosis, treatment, and prognosis in terms the patient can be reasonably expected to understand. When it is not medically advisable to give such information to the patient, the information should be made available to an appropriate person in his behalf. He has the right to know, by name, the physician responsible for coordinating his care.
3. The patient has the right to receive from his physician information necessary to give informed consent prior to the start of any procedure and/or treatment. Except in emergencies, such information for informed consent should include but not necessarily be limited to the specific procedure and/or treatment, the medically significant risks involved, and the probable duration of incapacitation. Where medically significant alternatives for care or treatment exist, or when the patient requests information concerning medical alternatives, the patient has the right to such information. The patient also has the right to know the name of the person responsible for the procedures and/or treatment.
4. The patient has the right to refuse treatment to the extent permitted by law and to be informed of the medical consequences of his action.
5. The patient has the right to every consideration of his privacy concerning his own medical care program. Case discussion, consultation, examination, and treatment are confidential and should be conducted discreetly. Those not directly involved in his care must have the permission of the patient to be present.

6. The patient has the right to expect that all communications and records pertaining to his care should be treated as confidential.
7. The patient has the right to expect that within its capacity a hospital must make reasonable response to the request of a patient for services. The hospital must provide evaluation, service, and/or referral as indicated by the urgency of the case. When medically permissible, a patient may be transferred to another facility only after he has received complete information and explanation concerning the needs for and alternatives to such a transfer. The institution to which the patient is to be transferred must first have accepted the patient for transfer.
8. The patient has the right to obtain information as to any relationship of his hospital to other health care and educational institutions insofar as his care is concerned. The patient has the right to obtain information as to the existence of any professional relationships among individuals, by name, who are treating him.
9. The patient has the right to be advised if the hospital proposes to engage in or perform human experimentation affecting his care or treatment. The patient has the right to refuse to participate in such research projects.
10. The patient has the right to expect reasonable continuity of care. He has the right to know in advance what appointment times and physicians are available and where. The patient has the right to expect that the hospital will provide a mechanism whereby he is informed by his physician or a delegate of the physician of the patient's continuing health care requirements following discharge.
11. The patient has the right to examine and receive an explanation of his bill regardless of source of payment.
12. The patient has the right to know what hospital rules and regulations apply to his conduct as a patient.

No catalog of rights can guarantee for the patient the kind of treatment he has a right to expect. A hospital has many functions to perform, including the prevention and treatment of disease, the education of both health professionals and patients, and the conduct of clinical research. All these activities must be conducted with an overriding concern for the patient, and, above all, the recognition of his dignity as a human being. Success in achieving this recognition assures success in the defense of the rights of the patient.

This policy document presents the official position of the American Hospital Association as approved by the Board of Trustees and House of Delegates.

During the 1970s the American Hospital Association's Board of Trustees had a Committee on Health Care for the Disadvantaged, which developed the *Statement on a Patient's Bill of Rights*. That document was approved by the AHA House of Delegates on February 6, 1973, and has been published in various forms. This reprinting and reclassification conforms with the current classification system for AHA documents. The contents are unchanged.

I
NAPNES Code of Ethics

Code of Ethics

The Licensed Practical/Vocational Nurse Shall

1. Consider as a basic obligation the conservation of life and the prevention of disease.
2. Promote and protect the physical, mental, emotional, and spiritual health of the patient and his family.
3. Fulfill all duties faithfully and efficiently.
4. Function within established legal guidelines.
5. Accept personal responsibility (for his/her acts) and seek to merit the respect and confidence of all members of the health team.
6. Hold in confidence all matters coming to his/her knowledge, in the practice of his profession, and in no way at no time violate this confidence.
7. Give conscientious service and charge just remuneration.
8. Learn and respect the religious and cultural beliefs of his/her patient and of all people.
9. Meet his/her obligation to the patient by keeping abreast of current trends in health care through reading and continuing education.
10. As a citizen of the United States of America, uphold the laws of the land and seek to promote legislation which shall meet the health needs of its people.

Reprinted with permission of the National Association for Practical Nurse Education and Service. Copyright 1988.

Index